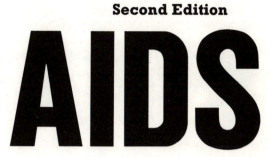

Second Edition

AIDS

The Acquired
Immune
Deficiency
Syndrome

Second Edition

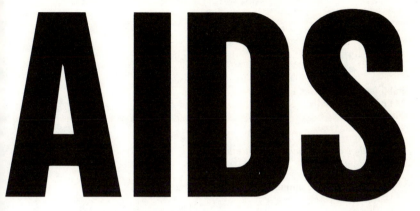

AIDS

The Acquired Immune Deficiency Syndrome

Dr. Victor G. Daniels
BSc, PhD, MB, BChir, Dip. Pharm. Med.

MTP PRESS LIMITED
a member of the KLUWER ACADEMIC PUBLISHERS GROUP
LANCASTER / BOSTON / THE HAGUE / DORDRECHT

Published in the UK and Europe by
MTP Press Limited
Falcon House
Lancaster, England

British Library Cataloguing in Publication Data

Daniels, Victor G.
    AIDS: the acquired immune deficiency syndrome.—2nd ed.
    1. AIDS (Disease)
    I. Title
    616.9′792   RC607.A26

    ISBN 0–7462–0035–8

Published in the USA by
MTP Press
A division of Kluwer Academic Publishers
101 Philip Drive
Norwell, MA 02061, USA

Library of Congress Cataloging in Publication Data

Daniels, Victor G.
    AIDS, the acquired immune deficiency
    syndrome—2nd ed.
    Bibliography: p.
    Includes index.
    1. AIDS (Disease)   I. Title.   [DNLM: 1. Acquired
Immunodeficiency Syndrome.   WD 308 D186a]
RC607.A26D36 1987   416.97′92   87–2651

    ISBN 0–7462–0035–8

Typeset and Printed by Butler & Tanner Ltd, Frome and London

Contents

Preface to the Second Edition

Within eighteen months of the preparation of the first edition much has happened in the AIDS field. The number affected are still increasing at an alarming rate – these are now (at December 1986) almost 30 000 cases in the United States and over 600 cases in the United Kingdom. Worldwide the AIDS pandemic is a most serious disease threat and now affects over 80 countries. It is estimated that for every AIDS patient there are about 50 other persons infected with the AIDS virus.

AIDS threatens every country and every society. The main preventative measures of health education to prevent the spread of AIDS must be taken by millions of individuals helped by governments and voluntary organizations. What is clear is that AIDS and AIDS-related conditions will be with us, in our hospitals and in our communities for many years to come.

It has been well established that the agent that causes AIDS is a virus called human immunodeficiency virus (HIV). People can catch HIV through sexual contact or by infected blood from infected needles and syringes, from infected mother to unborn child, or treatment with contaminated blood or blood products.

About 30 000 to 100 000 people in the United Kingdom and between 1 to 1.5 million in the United States are estimated to be infected with HIV. Clearly major health resources will be required since the long incubation period of AIDS (can be over 6 years from first infection) and the uncertainty of the number of infected people who will develop AIDS will produce many thousands of cases of AIDS within the next few years. Experts predict that anything from 30% to 100% of those infected with HIV will eventually develop fully expressed AIDS. In the United States, by 1991, forecasts have predicted about 270 000 cases of AIDS. In the United Kingdom by 1992 forecasts have suggested around 20 000 to 50 000 cases of AIDS.

I have taken the opportunity to update and where necessary revise the first edition. There are obviously many changes which I hope continue to satisfy the clear objective of this book to provide a comprehensive overview of all aspects of the disease. I am most grateful to all those who have helped me in the preparation of the second edition in particular my special thanks extend to Caroline Akehurst and David FitzSimons from the Bureau of Hygiene and Tropical Diseases who commented extensively on the first edition.

There is no doubt that AIDS will be the most significant event of our lifetime.

VICTOR G. DANIELS

Cambridge
January 1987

Preface to the First Edition

The acquired immune deficiency syndrome (AIDS) was first recognized only 5 years ago and has quickly attracted worldwide attention. The AIDS epidemic remains a phenomenon of unusual importance and an intense research effort is in progress throughout the world in an effort to understand the cause and develop treatment for this terrifying disease.

By January 1986 there were about 20 000 cases of AIDS worldwide; over 15 000 of these are in North America alone. AIDS appears to be increasing at an alarming rate. So far about 50% of these patients have died. Medical researchers and clinicians feel that the cases we see today represent only the tip of the iceberg and it appears that there will be more cases in the near future. The aim of this book, therefore, is to provide essential information for all those concerned with AIDS. This includes members of the general public including those at risk, public health workers and medical personnel, particularly general practitioners. It provides practical and reliable information on AIDS and avoids the sensational aspects of the disease. In this respect it allows the reader the opportunity to review the facts in full rather than as presented by the public media. The text offers guidance on the complex medical, social and sexual issues surrounding AIDS. The book has been written in a synoptic but readable style and contains many useful lists and tables that provide current information on AIDS. It is not a detailed textbook on the management of AIDS patients, rather it is a comprehensive overview of our present knowledge of all aspects of the disease.

In the preparation of this book I have consulted many sources of information including published articles in major medical journals.

Also I have made use of the various useful publications on AIDS published by the Terrence Higgins Trust, The Haemophilia Society and the Health Education Council. Some of the tables and figures on the incidence of AIDS were taken from the *Morbidity and Mortality Weekly Report* published by the Centers for Disease Control in Atlanta in the United States and the *Weekly Epidemiological Record* published by the World Health Organization.

I am grateful to the following people who helped me during the various stages of the preparation of the manuscript: Carol Connett who provided much of the early references and information; Dr Jacqueline Parkin from St Mary's Hospital, London, and Dr Marian McEvoy from the Communicable Disease Centre, London, for detailed comments and suggestions on the text; Prof Karol Sikora from the Hammersmith Hospital London, for his encouragement and scrutiny of the manuscript. My colleagues Drs Ian Scoular, Peter Crespin, Simon Barter and Will Tarbit read through and commented on several drafts of the manuscript. Andrew Rigg provided the finished diagrams. Finally, my thanks to my wife, Ruth, for her unfailing support and excellent proof reading and to Gill Norman who skilfully word-processed the text through its various stages.

To all of these, and others, I offer my grateful thanks and kindly acknowledge their help.

No book is without flaw and I would welcome suggestions that readers feel would make future editions more valuable.

VICTOR G. DANIELS

Cambridge
July 1985

Introduction

The acquired immune deficiency syndrome (AIDS) is a new and complicated disorder of the defence system of the body. AIDS attacks the sophisticated structure of immunity leaving the victim susceptible to organisms with which he had previously lived in relative harmony. These so-called opportunistic infections do not normally occur in healthy people. The breakdown in the immunological surveillance system in AIDS patients also predisposes the individual to the development of otherwise rare cancers such as Kaposi's sarcoma and lymphomas. The outstanding clinical feature of AIDS is the occurrence of opportunistic infections and cancer in previously healthy individuals. Opportunistic infections and cancer are mortal illnesses for the AIDS patient and the life expectancy for full-blown AIDS is about 2–3 years. In the last two years the cause of AIDS has been shown to be due to a virus called the human immuno-deficiency virus (HIV). This virus is capable of destroying a specific type of white blood cell called T-helper lymphocytes. Once the virus is 'caught' the victim harbours it for life. The body reacts against invasion of the AIDS virus by producing a specific antibody against the virus (HIV antibody). Unfortunately the antibody does not appear to neutralize the virus in the usual way and thus the individual may be infectious to others. Most people with HIV infection suffer little or no illness but some go on to develop fully-expressed AIDS. At present we do not understand the precise mechanisms of evolution of the disease whereby an HIV-positive individual develops AIDS. Certainly at the moment there is a large pool of HIV-positive individuals amongst the various risk groups – homosexuals, haemophiliacs, intravenous drug abusers – and only time will reveal what proportion of these people will go on to develop AIDS. The incubation period for the virus ranges from 6 months to 6 years or more with an average of around 28 months.

Individuals who have been infected with HIV can be classified into four general categories:

(1) Asymptomatic carriers – well with no signs of immuno-suppression.
(2) Persistent generalized lymphadenopathy (PGL) – well with glandular swellings (lymphadenopathy) in armpits, neck, groin etc.
(3) AIDS-related complex (ARC) – symptomatic with fatigue, fevers and often impairment of the immune system.
(4) Fully expressed AIDS – symptomatic with life-threatening opportunistic infections and Kaposi's sarcoma.

The treatment of AIDS is a challenge. So far there is no cure for AIDS – we only have treatment available for some of the complications of the disease. Development of an effective vaccine is currently under evaluation but it is thought that this will not be available for several years.

HOW TO USE THE BOOK

This book provides up-to-date information on AIDS and gives guidance on the various issues surrounding this disease. It is written in a synoptic non-sensational style and can be read by a wide audience.

Chapter 1 starts by discussing the prevalence and spread of the disease in terms of the distribution of the AIDS epidemic throughout the world. It contains numerous tables that serve to summarize the current situation.

Chapter 2 gives an account of the groups of individuals at risk of contracting AIDS – homosexuals, intravenous drug abusers, transfusion patients, children with AIDS etc. Each risk group is discussed in full in relation to the relative risks involved in contracting AIDS.

Chapter 3 presents critical new information on the cause of AIDS – the human immunodeficiency virus (HIV). Much of the first part of the chapter is technical and may be passed over quickly. The final sections provide an account of other factors involved in the development of AIDS.

Chapter 4 provides information on the transmission of the AIDS virus and discusses the various risks of sexual contact and transfer of the virus through blood and blood products.

Chapter 5 discusses the problem of testing for the AIDS virus (HIV) and what it means in clinical terms to be HIV antibody positive. Recommendations are also provided for individuals with HIV infection.

Chapter 6 presents information on early symptoms and signs of AIDS and provides descriptions of persistent generalized lymphadenopathy (PGL) and AIDS-related complex (ARC) which are thought to be precursors of fully-expressed AIDS.

Chapter 7 provides an account of the clinical picture of the disease and includes recent information on the definition of AIDS.

Chapter 8 discusses Kaposi's sarcoma in greater depth and may be passed over quickly if desired.

Chapter 9 concludes the main text of the book by reviewing the various treatment options available for AIDS, opportunistic infections of AIDS and AIDS-related Kaposi's sarcoma.

The appendices provide essential further information for those who seek amplification of the main text. A general background on viruses is provided to remind readers of the complexities of viral infection. A useful glossary is included in the appendices. There is a comprehensive appendix covering educational resources (pamphlets, books, addresses).

CHAPTER 1

Epidemiology of AIDS

AIDS is the most severe consequence of infection with the human immunodeficiency virus (HIV). It is invariably fatal.

THE EVOLUTION OF AIDS

The Acquired Immune Deficiency Syndrome (AIDS) appeared as if from nowhere in the Spring of 1981. AIDS apparently first appeared in 1979 and was brought to the attention of the medical community in 1981. *Acquired* means caught as opposed to inherited. *Immune deficiency* implies poor body defence mechanisms against infections and *syndrome* is a group of illnesses which helps to identify a particular disease – in this case AIDS. The first report of AIDS came from the Centers for Disease Control in Atlanta, Georgia (a public health body responsible for investigating epidemics and reports of new or unusual diseases), in the United States which described the cases of 5 young previously healthy homosexuals who had been treated in Los Angeles hospitals for a rare infection of the lungs – *Pneumocystis carinii* pneumonia (PCP). *Pneumocystis carinii* is a protozoan which parasitizes the lungs and as a result makes breathing very difficult. The opportunity for infection usually occurs only in individuals whose immune system is damaged or profoundly impaired. The unusual feature of these cases was, therefore, the occurrence of PCP in previously healthy individuals. Previously, this opportunistic infection had been almost exclusively associated with patients whose immune system was seriously impaired as a result of severe disease or drug therapy (for example those patients with severe congenital cellular immune deficiency, leukaemias, or those immunosuppressed as in renal transplantation). PCP was also recognized as a cause of fatal outbreaks of pneumonia in malnourished, sickly refugee children in Europe at the end of World War II.

At the same time in 1981 came reports of 26 previously healthy homosexuals in New York and California who had developed a severe form of a rare malignant cancer called Kaposi's sarcoma. Eight of these patients died within 24 months of diagnosis.

Kaposi's sarcoma is relatively common in equatorial Africa. In Europe and North America, however, it is restricted to elderly men of Mediterranean or Jewish ancestry. The occurrence of this rare tumour in men who were in the 20–40 years age range was therefore most unusual and of great concern.

The appearance of these two disorders *Pneumocystis carinii* pneumonia and Kaposi's sarcoma which had previously been restricted to well defined groups of individuals, but were now affecting previously fit younger men, suggested the occurrence of a new disease entity. The factor common to the new cases was that they all involved homosexuals. An additional feature was that the host response to these infections seemed to be impaired. It appeared that PCP and Kaposi's sarcoma were actually 'markers' of an underlying profound defect in the immune system. Since this immune deficiency was an acquired rather than inherited defect, the syndrome was termed the Acquired Immune Deficiency Syndrome, AIDS.

Why AIDS did not appear until the late 1970s is a scientific mystery but in the space of seven years AIDS has become epidemic throughout the Western world and throughout most parts of Africa.

TRACKING THE EPIDEMIC

Following on from the initial reports of AIDS, the Centers for Disease Control (CDC) in the United States set up a task force to detect the syndrome in the population and identify those at risk. Criteria for the definition of AIDS were drawn up based primarily on diagnosis of opportunistic infections and rare tumours in individuals with no evidence of immune suppression. The incidence of PCP could be monitored by reviewing requests made to the Centers for

Disease Control for pentamidine, an anti-protozoal drug used to treat this infection and available only from the Centers for Disease Control. Other opportunistic infections were monitored by written and telephone reports from health departments in the United States. In the United Kingdom the Communicable Disease Surveillance Centre (CDSC) of the Public Health Laboratory Service in London (who are responsible for National Epidemiological Surveillance) collects information about AIDS and issues a monthly analysis of statistics.

As surveillance got underway the epidemic nature of the outbreak was recognized with cases being reported not just in homosexuals but also, to a lesser extent, in intravenous drug abusers, haemophiliacs and Haitians.

By 1981 the number of AIDS cases in the United States had reached 337 including several reports of illness fitting the description of AIDS which had been documented as early as 1978. By December 1983, the total had risen to 4100 cases. Over 60% of these had died within the first year of diagnosis due to untreatable or overwhelming infections. By December 1984 the total was 7025; this had doubled to 14 049 by October 1985. In turn this figure had doubled to 28 098 (27 704 adults and 394 children by 8 December 1986 with doubling times of 9, 11 and 13 months. Of all reported cases 55% of the adults and 65% of the children are known to have died. About 79% of those patients diagnosed before January 1985 have died. Adult AIDS patients have been reported from all 50 states, the District of Columbia and 4 United States territories (see Figure 1.1).

Of 394 paediatric AIDS patients (at 8 Dec 1986) 347 (88%) are under 5 years of age, 57% are black, 22% Hispanic, 20% white. 311 cases come from families in which one or both parents had AIDS.

Regarding the United Kingdom the number of AIDS cases by comparison to the United States shows remarkably few on a per million population basis. The 1986 figure for the United States is 123 and for the United Kingdom 10.8. The percentage deaths in the groups are very similar; United States is 56.2% compared to about 48% in Britain (see Table 1.1).

In Europe 3735 cases had been reported to the World Health Organization (WHO) Collaborating Centre by September 1986. Table 1.2 shows the total number of AIDS cases and the estimated rates per million population. About 50% of these 3735 cases are known to have died. The highest rates per million population were

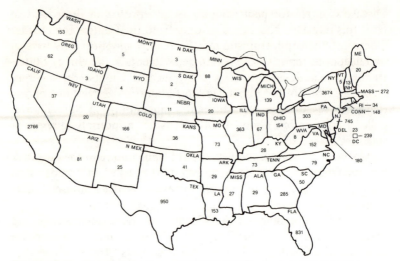

Figure 1.1   The distribution of 12 777 AIDS cases notified in the United States by 21 December 1985

observed in Switzerland: 26.2; Denmark 21.0; and Iceland 20.0. These rates are again relatively low by comparison with the United States. Belgium is in a special position because 56% of the notified cases are among Africans.

Worldwide no-one appears to be collecting the data and analysing the statistics. The WHO have details only for Europe, the CDSC concentrates on the British scene and the CDC monitors the United States. The number of world cases reported to the WHO as at 14 November 1986 is 34 448. Although this appears to be a large number of cases, to put this into perspective WHO have reported that in 1983 one million children died of malaria in Africa alone, while the organization estimated 50 million new cases of syphilis worldwide.

Overall since 1979 there has been a constant upward trend in the number of newly-diagnosed cases. There are no signs of the curve of incidence 'starting to bend' and it is difficult to predict when this will happen because the disease has a long incubation period. However, according to the Centers for Disease Control in Atlanta the rate of increase may have been levelling off since the middle of 1983. This probably reflects increasing awareness particularly among homo-sexuals of the risk of acquiring AIDS through multiple sexual part-

Table 1.1

AIDS in the United States[1]	Cases	Deaths
Pre 1981	76	63
1981	261	234
1982	999	853
1983	2 764	2 304
1984	5 531	4 251
1985	9 475	5 636
1986 to 29 December	9 897	2 960
Totals:	29 003	16 301

AIDS in Britain[2]	Cases	Deaths
1982	3	3
1983	26	26
1984	77	60
1985	165	87
1986	339	117
Totals:	610	293

[1] Source: Centers for Disease Control, Atlanta.
Total population of the United States is 237.5 million.
[2] Source: Department of Health
Figures are confirmed cases in the United Kingdom, where the total population is 56.4 million.

ners with consequent changes in lifestyle to minimize this risk. It may also be because a large proportion of the 'at risk' population has already been infected and those who are destined to develop AIDS have already got it, others have not and the pool of susceptible individuals is therefore less.

An epidemiologist Dr Marion McEvoy from the Communicable Disease Surveillance Centre in London reported in the *British Medical Journal* in February 1985 that the annual increase in AIDS cases in the United Kingdom 'Follows roughly an exponential rise … and if extrapolation is made to 1990 the estimated number of new cases is 10 000, but 95% confidence limits are 1 to 295 million'. However as pointed out by Dr McEvoy such predictions are not valid since the spread of an infectious disease is related to the number of susceptible people and as this number decreases the epidemic wanes. Other factors are also important; for example control measures and changes in sexual behaviour of at risk groups in limiting

Table 1.2 Total number of AIDS cases reported by 30 September 1986 in 27 European countries, and estimated rate per million population*

Country	Cases by 30 September 1986	Rates/ million
Austria	44	5.9
Belgium	180	18.2
Czechoslovakia	5	0.3
Denmark	107	21.0
Finland	14	2.9
France	1050	19.1
Germany, Federal Republic of	675	11.1
Greece	25	2.5
Iceland	4	20.0
Ireland	12	3.3
Israel	31	7.4
Italy	367	6.4
Luxembourg	5	12.5
Malta	5	12.5
Netherlands	180	12.4
Norway	26	6.2
Poland	1	0.0
Portugal	40	3.9
Romania	2	0.1
Spain	201	5.2
Sweden	76	9.2
Switzerland	170	26.2
United Kingdom	512	9.1
Yugoslavia	3	—
Total	3735	—

* German Democratic Republic, Hungary and the USSR have reported no cases; —, data not available.

the spread of the disease. Her projections for new cases in 1985 and 1986 were 144 and 336 and the actual figures were 165 and 337. Her projections continue: 785 in 1987 and 1837 in 1988.

More recent estimates have calculated in the UK that there could be an accumulative total of 20 000 to 50 000 cases of AIDS by 1992.

In the United States by 1991 forecasts suggest that the total number of cases of AIDS will be around 270 000.

Table 1.3 Reported cases of AIDS by state as of 8 September 1986 in the United States

State of residence*	Cases	% of total cases
California	5 545	22.7
Florida	1 615	6.6
New Jersey	1 496	6.1
New York	7 963	32.6
Other	7 833	32.0
Total	24 452	100.0

DISTRIBUTION OF THE AIDS EPIDEMIC

From the outset, the AIDS epidemic has shown marked geographical clustering of cases within the United States. The vast majority of patients have been associated with metropolitan areas on the east and west coasts, in particular New York City, and two cities in California, San Francisco and Los Angeles, and Florida. Together these areas have over 60% of AIDS cases (Table 1.3). This high incidence of AIDS is probably due to the congregation of large numbers of homosexuals in these cities and the fact that the 'fast lane' lifestyle in such communities includes:

(1) Group sexual practices and practices involving trauma to the rectal mucosa.
(2) Multiple sexual partners, which are thought to be important in the development of AIDS.

In addition New York City has one of the largest Haitian communities in the USA, an ethnic group which initially was thought to be at increased risk of developing AIDS. More likely this group of Haitians are at risk because of homosexuality and drug abuse and because it is a popular island for holidaying homosexuals from the United States. By 8 September 1986 the racial and ethnic breakdown of 24 102 AIDS cases was 60.4% white, 24.8% black, 14.2% Hispanic and 0.6% other but there were large variations in the risk groups.

Outside the United States, AIDS has been identified in all continents including most European and Scandinavian countries, Canada, Mexico, West Indies, South America, India and Africa, Australasia, Japan and Israel. The total number of cases worldwide by 14 Nov 1986 reported to WHO was 34 448.

The European experience in particular has mimicked the early American experience in that there has been a considerable increase in the number of AIDS cases. Generally, the same risk groups appear to be affected with the majority of patients being homosexual or bisexual men with a small proportion of drug abusers (Tables 1.4 and 1.5). Most of these early patients outside the United States (except Africa) probably contracted the disease through homosexual contacts in America, Europe or Haiti in the Caribbean.

Table 1.6 shows the proportion of AIDS patients by disease category. In the US the proportion of adult patients with Kaposi's sarcoma alone and with both Kaposi's sarcoma and *Pneumocystis carinii* pneumonia has decreased significantly from 1983 to April 1985. This is associated with a significant increase in the population of cases with *P. carinii* alone.

For comparison the incidence of Kaposi's sarcoma and opportunistic infections in the United States, United Kingdom and Europe is shown in Tables 1.6, 1.7a and 1.7b. The relatively small numbers in the UK make it impossible to draw any hard conclusions at this stage. But now more patients appear to have contracted the disease within the United Kingdom – probably as the pool of infection in this country increases AIDS will become more prevalent. It may be that any discrepancies that exist in the present data will disappear

Table 1.4 Distribution of adult AIDS cases by risk group in 27 European countries* 30 September 1986†

Risk group	Total	%
(1) Male homosexuals/bisexuals	2415	67
(2) IV drug addicts	421	12
(3) Haemophiliacs	137	4
(4) Transfusion recipients (without other risk factors)	81	2
(5) Groups 1 and 2	89	2
(6) No known risk factor – males	269	7
– females	132	4
(7) Unknown	83	2
Total	3627	100

* Austria, Belgium, Czechoslovakia, Denmark, Finland, France, Germany (Democratic Republic of), Germany (Federal Republic of), Greece, Hungary, Iceland, Ireland, Israel, Italy, Luxembourg, Malta, Netherlands, Norway, Poland, Portugal, Romania, Spain, Sweden, Switzerland, United Kingdom, USSR and Yugoslavia.
† Excludes 108 paediatric AIDS cases.

once the number of AIDS cases in Britain reaches a similar order of magnitude as the cases in the United States.

The first reported case in the United Kingdom in December 1981 was a 49-year-old homosexual in Bournemouth who presented with AIDS nine months after returning from Miami. One of the earliest of the British cases reported to die with AIDS was Terrence Higgins in 1982. A trust has been set up in his name that provides advice and support to those in need. In 1982 in Britain a surveillance scheme was set up to monitor AIDS based on reports by genito-urinary physicians, other clinicians, laboratory reports of opportunistic infections and death certification of AIDS and Kaposi's sarcoma. Few further cases occurred until the end of 1983 when the numbers rose from 13 (June) to 29 (December). At least two-thirds of the first 31 cases reported by January 1984 had had American sexual partners and the majority of the homosexual patients live in London. Further details of the United Kingdom AIDS patients are shown in Table 1.8. As of December 1986 610 cases have been reported in the

Table 1.5 AIDS patients by patient group, United States of America, to 8 December 1986

Patient group	Cases			
	Male	*Female*	*Total*	*%*
Adult				
Homosexual/bisexual	18162	—	18162	65.6
IV drug user	3760	963	4723	17.0
Homosexual/bisexual				
and IV drug user	2165	—	2165	7.8
Haemophilia patient	233	7	240	0.9
Heterosexual contact[1]	542	514	1056	3.8
Transfusion recipient	324	181	505	1.8
Other/unknown[2]	648	205	853	3.1
Total	25834	1870	27704	100.0
Paediatric (aged under 13)				
Parent with AIDS or at increased risk for AIDS			311	79
Haemophilia patient			22	6
Transfusion recipient			51	13
Other/unknown			10	3
Total			394	100.0
TOTAL			28098	100.0

[1]Includes 485 persons (81 men, 404 women) who have had heterosexual contact with a person with AIDS or at risk for AIDS and 571 persons (461 men, 110 women) without other identified risks who were born in countries in which heterosexual transmission is believed to play a major role.
[2]Includes patients on whom risk information is incomplete.

Table 1.6   Percentage distribution of adult AIDS patients by disease and date of report, United States of America, to 8 December 1986

Disease	Before May 1983	May 1983– April 1984	May 1984– April 1985	Total to Dec 86
Kaposi's sarcoma	24.7	24.1	18.9	15
Kaposi's sarcoma and P. carinii pneumonia	10.3	6.7	4.3 ⎫	
P. carinii pneumonia, no Kaposi's sarcoma	51.3	51.7	59.5 ⎬	64
Other opportunistic diseases	13.7	17.5	17.2	21
Total	100.0	100.0	100.0	100

Table 1.7a   Surveillance of AIDS in the United Kingdom: October 1986

	Cases	(%)	Deaths
Kaposi's sarcoma	115	(21.0)	37
P. carinii pneumonia	247	(45.1)	136
Kaposi's sarcoma and P. carinii pneumonia	41	(7.5)	18
Other opportunistic infections	135	(24.6)	82
Cerebral lymphoma*	2	(0.4)	2
Non-Hodgkin's lymphoma	8	(1.5)	3
Total	548	(100.0)	278

* Cerebral lymphoma is a rare tumour that occurs in AIDS patients

Table 1.7b   Surveillance of AIDS in Europe: 30 September 1986

	Cases	(%)	Deaths
Kaposi's sarcoma	644	(17.2)	188
Opportunistic infections (OI)	2561	(68.6)	1370
OIs and Kaposi's sarcoma	430	(11.5)	251
Other	100	(2.7)	56
Total	3735	(100.0)	1865

United Kingdom; 293 of these patients have died. Of the 610 reported cases, 538 (88%) of them were homosexual or bisexual men. There were 14 cases in heterosexual risk groups, 25 men with haemophilia and 1 case in no known risk group (see Table 1.8). The geographic distribution of these cases shows that about 77% have been reported

Table 1.8 Cumulative totals of UK reports of AIDS cases, by transmission characteristics, to 31 December 1986

Transmission characteristic	Number of cases			%	Number of deaths
	Male	*Female*	*Total*		
Homosexual/bisexual	538	—	538	88.2	244
Intravenous drug abuser (IVDA)	7	2	9	1.5	2
Homosexual and IVDA	6	—	6	1.0	4
Haemophiliac	25	—	25	4.1	19
Recipient of blood: abroad	3	3	6	1.0	5
UK	3	1	4	0.6	4
Heterosexual:					
presumed infected abroad	9	5	14	2.3	9
presumed infected in UK	1	3	4	0.6	3
Child of HIV antibody positive mother	1	2	3	0.5	2
Other	—	1	1	0.2	1
Totals	593	17	610	100	293

from the four Thames regions. AIDS therefore appears to be confined to a recognized risk group in the United Kingdom and is very similar to the United States AIDS patients – about 73% of all American cases are homosexual or bisexual men (see Table 1.5). But only 48% of 4758 identified carriers of HIV antibodies were reported in the four Thames regions, with over 18% in Scotland. However the real total of carriers is thought to be much higher.

In the United States reported cases have increased substantially in all patient groups. Since 1981 to April 1985 the proportion of AIDS cases in transfusion recipients has increased significantly but has steadied at about 2% by August 1986. Among the 394 AIDS patients under 13, about 79% came from families in which one or both parents had AIDS or were at risk of developing AIDS; about 13% had received transfusions of blood or blood products and about 6% had haemophilia.

The seriousness of the AIDS epidemic is illustrated by the fact that in New York and San Francisco death from AIDS is as common as death from cancer or heart disease and several times more common than death from road traffic accidents.

The distribution of the European AIDS cases by risk group shows that 70% of cases are homosexuals or bisexuals including 2% who are also intravenous drug abusers. About 12% of cases are drug abusers only and about 2% of cases are associated with the use of blood products. Haemophiliacs account for about 4% of all cases (see Table 1.4).

So far the growth rate of AIDS in Europe is similar to that of the United States but appears to be trailing three years behind. Whether AIDS in Europe will reach a growth rate similar to that observed in America is obviously a matter for concern. However, wide media coverage of the AIDS situation in the United States has brought the disease to the early attention of the European public and will hopefully lead to a stabilization in the growth rate. This change in the incidence of new cases may be the result in the United States of changes in lifestyle in the risk groups. However the development of new cases depends on the length of incubation of the AIDS virus. Some studies have suggested that it may take up to six years or more after infection before clinical signs become apparent and the number of individuals who develop fully-expressed AIDS will, of course, depend upon the initial infection rate.

Early in 1985 in the United Kingdom new measures were introduced by the British Government to control the spread of AIDS. In October 1985 the screening of blood donors in the United Kingdom for HIV antibodies was introduced. Late in 1986 the government launched a £20 million publicity campaign, using the media, including TV, and the distribution of leaflets to all 23 million households. The Government stopped short of making AIDS a notifiable disease since they considered that the condition was being effectively monitored. However, it was felt that there might be 'very rare and exceptional cases' where a patient was dangerously infective that powers would be sought to detain him in hospital. The main objective of notification of a disease is to enable rapid preventive action to be taken when appropriate to bring the disease under control. It is the legal duty of the clinician to notify the local medical officer for environmental health, who may be the district community physician in England, Wales or the chief administrative medical officer in Scotland, if he suspects that his patient is suffering from a notifiable disease. The clinician may notify by telephone but he is also required to provide a written certificate. The list of notifiable infectious diseases in England and Wales is shown in Table 1.9.

Table 1.9 Notifiable infectious diseases, England and Wales 1981

Acute encephalitis	Leprosy	Scarlet fever
Acute meningitis	Leptospirosis	Smallpox
Acute poliomyelitis	Malaria	Tetanus
Anthrax	Marburg disease	Tuberculosis
Cholera	Measles	Typhoid fever
Diphtheria	Ophthalmia	Typhus fever
Dysentery	neonatorum	Viral haemorrhagic
Food poisoning	Paratyphoid fever	fever
Infective jaundice	Plague	Whooping cough
Lassa fever	Rabies	Yellow fever
	Relapsing fever	

Note: There are minor differences in Scotland and Northern Ireland.

UK PUBLIC HEALTH REGULATIONS AS THEY RELATE TO THE SPREAD OF AIDS

The Public Health (Infectious Diseases) Regulations 1985 make available provisions to control the spread of AIDS. The Regulations make the disease subject to certain provisions of the 1984 Act that already operate in respect of other infectious diseases. They are intended for use in very exceptional circumstances only. They allow for medical examination, removal to hospital and detention there of patients in a dangerously infectious state and will be used if ever the necessity should arise. The Regulations will also allow restrictions to be placed on the handling of bodies of AIDS sufferers. The provisions of the Public Health (Control of Disease) Act 1984 applied by the Public Health (Infectious Diseases) Regulations 1985 are as follows:

(1) To allow a local authority, with the consent of the appropriate health authority, to make an application to a Justice of the Peace for an order to remove a person suffering from AIDS to hospital where there is a risk to others (Section 37 of the 1984 Act).

(2) To allow a local authority to make an application to a Justice of the Peace to have an AIDS patient detained in hospital where other suitable precautions will be taken to prevent the spread of the diseases (Section 38 of the 1984 Act).

(3) To allow a Justice of the Peace to make an order for a person

believed to be suffering from AIDS to be medically examined by a registered medical practitioner (Section 35 of the 1984 Act).

(4) To place restrictions on the removal of a body of an AIDS sufferer from hospital (Section 43 of the 1984 Act).

(5) To require all reasonably practicable steps to be taken to prevent persons unnecessarily coming into contact with, or proximity to, the body of an AIDS sufferer (Section 44 of the 1984 Act).

The government's advertising campaign to contain the spread of the AIDS virus started in the Spring of 1986. Advertisements were placed in national newspapers and in gay and contact press in March and April 1986. At this time there were already 300 cases of AIDS in the UK. A market research survey showed that the government's initial public education strategy indicated that one quarter of a sample of 1400 adults aged 18–64 years had been aware of this campaign.

A further health education campaign has been mounted more recently. A leaflet called '*AIDS: Don't Die of Ignorance*' was distributed in January 1987 to all 23 million households in the UK. At the same time extensive newspaper advertising and a bill-board poster campaign at 1500 street locations was initiated. This was complemented by national and local radio commercials as well as television advertisements. In addition advertising in 1200 cinemas throughout the country has been used. Only time will tell if this extensive media coverage costing in excess of £20 million will help to stem the spread of the AIDS virus.

To a modest extent some changes are already visible – a MORI poll published by *The Times* showed that as a result of the information campaign about 42% of married people said that they would be less likely to have extra-marital sex, and 26% of young single people are more likely to use a condom. The poll, conducted amongst a representative quota sample of 1093 adults aged 18 to 54 at 55 constituency sampling points throughout Britain, also revealed a clear understanding of how AIDS is transmitted. There were hints of panic behind some responses; 16% said they were less likely to give blood, 39% were less likely to give mouth-to-mouth resuscitation to strangers, 22% would not help a stranger injured in an accident. Also about 30% of respondents with children under 18 would decline to send their children to a school where another child had AIDS.

CHAPTER 2

Who can get AIDS? – the risk groups

Strictly speaking almost anyone could develop AIDS if exposed to infected blood or blood products; however the epidemic in the United States has highlighted some individuals who are at a greater risk of acquiring the disease:

(1) Homosexual or bisexual men
(2) Intravenous drug abusers who share hypodermic needles
(3) Haemophiliacs who have received infected blood products
(4) Transfusion patients who have received infected blood products
(5) Heterosexual partners of AIDS patients or those infected with human immunodeficiency virus (HIV)
(6) Infants of parents with AIDS
(7) Cases associated with central Africa
(8) Haitians

The reason why these particular groups have been affected is probably a reflection of the mode of transmission of the infection and provides some clues as to the causative agent or agents involved.

(1) HOMOSEXUAL OR BISEXUAL MEN

Outside Africa, men account for 90–95% of AIDS cases and about two-thirds of these men have been homosexuals or bisexuals. In some parts of the San Francisco homosexual community the risk of contracting AIDS is thought to be about 1 per 350 inhabitants. However, taking the United States as a whole less than 1 per 1000 homosexual men have become AIDS patients. In Great Britain the exact figures are not known but estimates put the present risk at roughly 10 per million of the population or 1 out of every 2000 British homosexuals. It is very difficult to make accurate predictions since only by following risk groups over a considerable length of time can reliable data be obtained.

Approximately 90% of homosexual men with AIDS have been aged between 20 and 49 years at the time of diagnosis and come from all major racial groups in the United States.

The risk of contracting AIDS in homosexuals is thought to be associated with exposure to semen or blood during anal intercourse and with multiple or anonymous casual partners (greater than 50 partners per year). In a survey of male homosexuals with Kaposi's sarcoma in the United States, 50% had had 10 or more different sexual partners a month compared to about 17% of healthy homosexual men questioned. The number of sexual partners reported by homosexuals ranges from 1 to over 1000 a year.

Infection by the putative AIDS agent within the homosexual population indicates that close intimate contact usually by penetrating anal intercourse is required for transmission of the AIDS agent. It is also related to the use of illicit drugs and a greater history of sexually transmitted diseases and generally though not always associated with the 'fast-track' lifestyle of some homosexuals.

The Terrence Higgins Trust (Tel. 01-833 2971), a registered charity set up to inform, advise and help on AIDS, offers the following advice to homosexuals on how to reduce the risk of getting AIDS.

(a) Have sex with fewer men.
(b) Avoid anal sex, except possibly with your regular partner(s).
(c) Avoid sex with men who have had sex in high risk areas (especially in the United States) in the last three years.
(d) Have sex with men who have few other sexual partners.
(e) Since the putative AIDS agent has been found in saliva, perhaps the only safe sex is mutual masturbation, body rubbing and dry kissing.
(f) Homosexuals should not give blood or carry an organ donor card.

Anal sex is, of course, a high-risk activity and the Trust advise that condoms should be used with a water-based lubricant like KY jelly or Duragel.

More specific guidelines for safer sex are given on page 119.

The Terrence Higgins Trust operates on several levels, offering those at risk and the general public a variety of services, including:

(a) Counselling groups who are responsible for the telephone service. These groups also provide support for people with AIDS and those people who have been exposed to the putative AIDS agent. 'Buddies' are a non-medical home care team that provide a supportive relationship for patients with AIDS. They deal with practical problems such as incontinence, meals on wheels, the DHSS etc.

(b) Education
    (i) Information to the general public through publications.
    (ii) Information to professionals through publications.
    (iii) Education to the risk groups through publications and visits to gay pubs and clubs in and outside London, informing of sex risks and discussing safer sexual practices.

Quite what effect the Trust will have on the sexual and social behaviour of gays remains to be determined. It is still early days. Reports from the United States have suggested that many homosexual men are using condoms during anal–genital intercourse and have reduced their number of different sexual partners. However a recent study in 1985 in America has shown that homosexuals who have been identified as a key risk group for several years are still donating blood. The survey showed that of 200 homosexuals 20 had donated a total of 36 units of blood between 1982 and 1984. More recently this figure has dropped significantly and fewer gays are donating blood.

There has been in the UK an encouragingly sharp decrease in the incidence of gonorrhoea and syphilis in homosexual men and, doubtless, gay men have made substantial changes to their lifestyle.

(2) INTRAVENOUS DRUG ABUSERS

It is thought there are about 60 000 to 150 000 people in the UK who regularly misuse drugs by the intravenous route.

Among heterosexual men or women with AIDS in the United States, approximately 64% are reported to be users of intravenous (IV) drugs especially heroin and cocaine. The drugs themselves are not the cause of AIDS. More than 6000 heroin users in Britain are unaffected by the syndrome. However, the needles used to inject the drugs are often shared by several addicts and intravenous drug users 'rent' needles in so-called 'shooting galleries'. 'Booting' or the repeated withdrawal and injection of blood into the syringe may increase the risk of transmission of the AIDS agent. An infectious agent may easily be transmitted by using blood-contaminated needles to inject drugs in a similar way to the transmission of hepatitis B (see later). Frequent needle sharing with many individuals is analogous to the high rate of sexual activity among some homosexuals. AIDS victims in this group in the United States have been shown to be of a lower socioeconomic status than the homosexual male group and have a different geographical distribution; approximately 67% came from the New York–New Jersey area compared with 38% of the homosexual men (see Table 1.3).

In drug addicts, studies have shown that the prevalence of anti-bodies to the AIDS agent has varied from 6% in parts of the United Kingdom to 87% in parts of the United States. In Italy and Spain the prevalence is about 50–57% and it is thought that this is linked in all countries to the length of the history of drug addiction.

It is thought that about 50% of intravenous drug abusers in Edinburgh have antibodies to HIV and is attributed to the high frequency of needle and equipment ('works') sharing found in the city. Several clinics in the city operate a 'swop-shop' arrangement whereby old needles and syringes are exchanged for new. This system works well in Holland and the British Government are to extend the policy to cover several other major cities in the United Kingdom.

The following recommendations (taken from the Scottish Committee on HIV Infection and Intravenous Drug Misuse (1986)) should be observed to prevent the further spread of HIV in intravenous drug abusers:

(1) Injecting drug misusers who cannot or will not abstain from misuse must be educated in safer drug-taking practices. It is of the utmost importance that those who continue to inject are persuaded to use clean equipment and never to share it. Clean equipment should therefore not be denied to those who cannot be dissuaded from injection. In this connection authorities should be reminded that threat to life of the spread of HIV infection is greater than that of drug misuse. On balance, the prevention of

spread should take priority over any perceived risk of increased drug misuse.

(2) Practitioners should be informed that it may be an appropriate part of the management of individual patients, in the interests of limiting the spread of infection, to issue needles and syringes and that this should be done on a one-for-one exchange basis for a needle and syringe. This should be linked with a simple reminder to practitioners that tests for drugs in the urine which can be used in the surgery are available and with the warning that any drugs which were being given to the patient could be crushed up and injected. Testing for HIV antibodies, with appropriate pre-counselling, should be offered to those who are given this equipment.

(3) Substitution prescription should be considered for those patients for whom it is judged that it will assist in reducing or stopping injection. It should also be considered as a means of establishing and maintaining effective contact with injecting drug misusers.

(4) All drug misusers must be given advice on 'safe sex' with particular emphasis on the use of condoms. Family Planning advice should be readily available, linked to counselling about the grave risk to an infant born to infected parents.

A health education campaign similar to 'safe sex' (see later) is required to promote 'safe shooting' to halt the spread of HIV among the drug abusing community.

(3) HAEMOPHILIACS

The development of AIDS in haemophiliacs in the United States was first reported in 1982. By 8 December 1986 a total of 240 haemophiliacs have been the victims of AIDS in the United States out of a population of about 20 000 Americans affected with this blood disorder. This represents a prevalence of about 1.2%. None of these people are reported to be homosexual or fit into any other risk category for AIDS (see Table 1.5).

In Britain, by December 1986, the frequency of haemophiliacs with AIDS was slightly lower; only twenty-five haemophiliacs out of a total population of 4500 haemophiliacs receiving treatment have so far developed AIDS. This represents a prevalence of about 0.55%.

In the absence of any obvious risk factor in this group of AIDS patients, most attention has been given to the clotting factors as a likely source of transmission. Haemophiliacs suffer from an inherited defect in the blood clotting mechanism in which one or two of the clotting factors essential for clot formation are missing. As a result, even minor wounds may cause a haemophiliac to bleed to death. This genetically-determined (sex-linked recessive) disorder is expressed only in men, although women can be carriers of this trait. To live a reasonably normal life, haemophiliacs must receive regular injections of the missing clotting factors. These are most commonly factor VIII although factor IX or even both of these may occasionally be required. Deficiency of factor VIII is the commonest disorder and is sometimes referred to as haemophilia A. Deficiency of factor IX is sometimes referred to as haemophilia B or Christmas disease after the surname of a Canadian patient. The aim of treatment is to provide replacement of the clotting factors. The materials available for this purpose are cryoprecipitate and freeze-dried (lyophilized) concentrate. Cryoprecipitate is made by slow thawing of frozen plasma (at 4°C) which leaves a residue rich in factor VIII. Lyophilized concentrate is derived from about 2000–5000 different donors while cryoprecipitate is derived from a smaller pool of about 20 donors.

Huge numbers of plasma donations (several thousands) are required to manufacture the factor VIII and IX concentrates. Thus a person with severe haemophilia may, therefore, be exposed to tens of thousands of donors each year. If any one of these donors is an AIDS carrier then the AIDS agent causing immune deficiency may be transmitted in the donated blood. Haemophiliacs are as a result far more at risk from contracting AIDS than recipients of other blood transfusions where relatively few donors are involved. At the present time the risk of AIDS in United Kingdom haemophiliacs is around 1 in 200 (see Table 2.1). The risk from blood transfusion has been put at around 1 in 100 000 or less, but this can also vary a great deal (see later). AIDS is now the most important complication of treatment for haemophilia.

All twenty-five of the United Kingdom haemophiliacs who developed AIDS received factor VIII concentrate from America. At present, about 60% of the factor VIII concentrate now used in the United Kingdom comes from America. It is estimated that British production should be self-sufficient within the next year or so. Although no cases of AIDS have so far appeared in recipients of

Table 2.1 Haemophilia and AIDS

	Total population	Total AIDS cases	Haemophiliacs with AIDS	Haemophiliac population requiring treatment
United States of America[1]	237 million	29 003	269	20 000
United Kingdom[2]	56 million	610	25	4 500

[1] Data at 29 December 1986
[2] Data at 31 December 1986

factor VIII concentrates from British plasma, it has been reported that antibodies to the AIDS agent are appearing in patients treated with locally produced plasma.

Some other excellent news was the announcement in mid 1984 from the Royal Free Hospital, Speywood Laboratories and the biotechnology company Genentech in San Francisco that the gene for factor VIII has been isolated and cloned. Factor VIII has been synthesized in mammalian cell-culture. It is thought that synthetic factor VIII should be available for use by haemophiliacs some time towards the end of the 1980s. Clearly this method of production would provide a hepatitis- and AIDS-free therapeutic product.

Irrespective of where factor VIII is obtained, however, the problem of how to reduce the risk of contracting AIDS by haemophiliacs and other recipients of blood products remains. The situation unfortunately is not likely to alter until a definite blood test for the AIDS agent is developed for screening donated blood and diagnosing the infection.

Heat treatment of blood products in the same way as pasteurization of milk helps to reduce contamination by infective agents and so reduces the risk of transmitting the AIDS agent. However heat treatment usually at a temperature of around 60°C reduces the biological activity of the clotting factors. Whole blood cannot be warmed above body temperature since the red and white blood cells are destroyed by heat. The Centers for Disease Control in the United States have tested the effect of heat treatment on viruses (including the AIDS virus) added to factor VIII concentrate and confirm that heat treatment reduces viral contamination. They concluded that 'Preliminary evidence concerning the effects of heat treatment on the viability of the AIDS virus is strongly supportive of the usefulness of heat treatment in reducing the potential for transmission of the AIDS virus in factor concentrate products and suggest that the use of non-heat-treated factor concentrates should be limited.'

There is as yet no agreed standard for treating plasma products. Temperatures vary between 60°C and 69°C and duration from 10 to 72 hours. The *Lancet* in 1986 reported two suspected cases of HIV infection that occurred after receiving heat-treated Factor VIII. It thus seems possible that some virus could be left after heat treatment particularly if the preparation is treated at a lower temperature and/or for a shorter time.

Obviously the cost of producing heat-treated concentrate is more since there is a loss in yield of clotting factor by heating. But the benefit of such a product both to the patients and society as a whole well outweighs the cost.

Apart from heat treatment the only option available to reduce the risk of AIDS being transmitted by blood products is to exclude donors who belong to groups at high risk for developing AIDS. In Britain, where blood donation is voluntary, the DHSS has prepared a leaflet for the National Blood Transfusion Service called 'AIDS Important Information for Blood Donors'. The leaflet asks donors not to give blood if they think they may either have the disease or be at risk from it (see Appendix 2).

The Haemophilia Society (123 Westminster Bridge Road, London SE1 7HR) have offered the following advice to prevent transmission of the AIDS agent from potentially infected haemophiliac patients to their sexual partners, immediate household members and offspring.

(a) Use of a condom or sheath along with a spermicidal lubricant during sexual intercourse.
(b) Some haemophilia centres are advising that its patients should think very carefully before having children, for the time being.
(c) Exercise extreme care in preparing and clearing up when a relative helps with a factor VIII infusion.
(d) Sexual partners are advised not to give blood nor carry an organ donor card.
(e) Haemophiliacs are also advised to keep their toothbrushes separate in case of a bleed.

This advice is obviously very sensible though it may cause some embarrassment and inconvenience amongst haemophiliacs. Some recent work from Dr Richard Tedder at the Middlesex Hospital in

London has demonstrated a rising incidence in antibodies to the AIDS agent in haemophiliacs over the past five years or so.

A study in Newcastle in 1985 found antibodies to HIV in three out of 36 sexual partners of patients with severe haemophilia A. For two of these women no other risk factors were identified.

A study in Denmark in 1985 demonstrated that heterosexual transmission of the AIDS agent can occur between haemophiliacs and sexual partners. This case was a 17-year-old girl who practised oral, vaginal and anal intercourse with her haemophiliac friend. It was suggested that infection with the AIDS agent may be facilitated by the practice of anal intercourse as it appears to be in homosexual men.

The development of heat-treatment and other modifications in the manufacture of blood clotting factors along with the introduction of universal donor screening has virtually eliminated the risk of HIV transmission by this route.

A fuller account of blood products and the putative AIDS agent is given in Chapter 5.

(4) OTHER RECIPIENTS OF BLOOD PRODUCTS

Blood products other than those used in the treatment of hae-mophilia have also been associated with AIDS. As of December 1986 there have been 505 cases of possible transfusion-associated AIDS in the United States and this group accounts for about 2.0% of all reported cases of AIDS (see Table 1.5). So far in the United Kingdom there have been ten reported cases of transfusion-related AIDS (see Table 1.8). Further it is known that blood has been donated in the United Kingdom by a man in Wessex with AIDS. In this case all recipients of his blood and blood plasma have been traced and include thirty-nine patients, thirty-six with haemophilia. No patient has, so far, developed AIDS and all patients will be closely monitored for the development of antibody to the AIDS agent.

Transfusion-related AIDS patients have been identified by the following criteria:

(a) No other known risk factor for developing AIDS.

(b) Medical history includes transfusions of blood or blood products (packed cells, plasma, platelets, whole blood) within 5 years preceding the diagnosis of AIDS.

One of the most convincing and widely recognized transfusion related cases occurred in a 20-month-old male infant from San Francisco. He developed a syndrome virtually identical to the AIDS seen in adults following a blood transfusion. Tracing of blood donors showed that one of the 19 donors was a 48-year-old man who was well at the time of donation but who subsequently died of AIDS. A similar case involving four Australian neonates who died after receiving blood donated by an AIDS sufferer has further confirmed this route of transmission. In other cases of transfusion-associated AIDS, some of the donors traced have belonged to groups at high risk of contracting AIDS although showing no symptoms of the syndrome. Early in 1985 in the United Kingdom a baby aged 21 months died after contracting AIDS. The child was born in America at 26 weeks into the pregnancy and after birth he developed several complications including a heart complaint which necessitated intensive care and multiple blood transfusions. Later on the boy was admitted to a hospital in England with pneumonia and severe weight loss. He did not respond to medical treatment and eventually he died. It was thought that the child had received infected blood in the United States.

Some evidence has suggested that exposure to as little as one unit of blood may cause infection. However, given the small number of suspected cases of AIDS in this group, it is generally agreed that the risk of not accepting a needed blood transfusion far outweighs the risk of contracting AIDS from transfused blood. Calculated on the basis of an estimated ten million units of blood given each year in the United States, the frequency of transfusion associated AIDS during the last 5 years is about 1 case in 100 000, i.e. a relatively low but nevertheless worrying risk. However certain patients such as those undergoing heart surgery or those with haematological disorders, e.g. acute leukaemia, may receive whole blood, platelet transfusions, cryoprecipitate or other blood products from over 50 donors. Before screening for HIV was introduced it is thought that the risk in these patients may be as high as 1 in 200 in certain areas of Britain.

Doctors from St Thomas's Hospital in London have suggested

that self-donation of blood (autologous transfusion) would minimize the risk of catching AIDS. Anyone due for elective surgery, provided they are not anaemic, may safely give units of blood in the period leading up to the operation. At operation, if blood is required, the patient then receives his own blood. This practice has been advocated by the American Association of Blood Banks and the American Red Cross since 1983. Blood donation stimulates sites of red blood cell production – the bone marrow – to make more red blood cells. Autotransfusion is especially useful in those operations where the patient may lose a great deal of blood, for example in heart and orthopaedic surgery.

Blood donors in the United States are now being asked to agree to samples of their blood being stored so that when a screening test for AIDS does become available, these samples can be tested. Meanwhile, recipients of blood are being followed up so that the proportion of those given infected blood who then acquire the disease can be determined. Obviously, this involves enormous ethical problems, for example, should recipients of blood found later to be infected be told, and, further, should donors who are found to be carriers be informed?

As at January 1987, in the UK it is clear that donors in high risk groups have been responsive to the advice not to give blood since only 65 of more than three million donations have proved positive for HIV antibodies. On questioning, most of those found to be positive were male homosexuals who had misunderstood the advice given by the DHSS. Only four anti-HIV positive donors denied being in one of the high-risk categories. The risk of donations containing undetectable AIDS virus was put at 'about one in a million'.

People who should *not* give blood or plasma:

(a) Sexual contacts of people with AIDS.
(b) Men who have had homosexual contact.
(c) Bisexual men (as above) and their heterosexual partners.
(d) Sexual contacts of people receiving multiple blood transfusions, including haemophiliacs.
(e) Present or former drug addicts who have injected themselves and their heterosexual partners.
(f) People who have arrived or returned from Zaire or surrounding countries in East and Central Africa, or from Haiti in the last few years, and their sexual partners. This applies to those 'risk

groups' who have had blood transfusions, drug injections and sexual contact there etc.

The development of universal donor screening and requests to high risk groups not to donate blood has virtually eliminated the likelihood of HIV infection as a result of receiving blood products. A fuller account of blood products and the putative AIDS agent is given in Chapter 5.

(5) HETEROSEXUAL PARTNERS OF AIDS PATIENTS

A most striking epidemiological feature of AIDS is its failure so far to spread widely in the community. Only limited spread to female sexual contacts has been reported. This is quite unlike the picture of the usual sexually transmitted diseases. Fully-expressed AIDS or severe immune deficiency has been reported in the female sexual partners of patients with AIDS. In the United States the proportion of women affected has remained constant at about 7% of all cases.

A number of studies have suggested that AIDS may be transmitted heterosexually. In the majority of these cases women have reported sexual relationships with either male AIDS cases or with men who belonged to the AIDS risk group. The role of anal–genital intercourse in the development of AIDS in females has so far not been studied.

A preliminary study in America has shown that transmission of the putative AIDS agent occurs between haemophiliacs and their heterosexual partners. Only two wives of haemophiliacs out of a study group of 21 wives were positive for antibody against the AIDS agent. The agent may not have been transmitted sexually but the authors concluded that longitudinal follow-up of these cases will show whether additional wives will develop antibodies to the AIDS agent. There is however still the worrying possibility of heterosexual spread of the disease outside the usual risk groups.

At the recent International AIDS Conference in Atlanta in the Spring of 1985 a researcher, Dr Robert Redfield, reported that nearly a third of the 41 AIDS patients being studied at the Walter Reed Hospital in Washington (The American Armies Medical Institute) had not been exposed to high risk groups such as homosexuals or intravenous drug abusers. The common epidemiological factors in this group of patients included more than 100 heterosexual contacts over the past five years including prostitutes. The United States

Pentagon has organized a series of special radio warnings to American troops in Europe warning them that female prostitutes are a potential reservoir of the AIDS virus. The Pentagon however has no current plans to declare certain red-light districts out of bounds because this has never worked in the past. However in January 1986 the British Army declared the coastal strip of Kenya around Mombasa out of bounds to UK troops exercising in Kenya. The troops were also issued with a free supply of condoms.

Against this background extensive dissemination of the virus could occur from the sexual activities of male intravenous drug abusers and bisexual males – it is thought that about 10–15% of homosexual men are bisexual. These so-called bridge groups may spread the virus from the present high-risk groups into low-risk groups. Their female sexual partners therefore constitute a potentially high risk group and in many instances may be unaware of their infectivity.

Spread of infection from female to male has also been observed. One case history from the United States underlines the seriousness of this route of infection. A bisexual man with AIDS infected his wife who had no other known risk factors. The husband died as a result of AIDS and his wife not knowing of her infection with HIV moved in with her next-door neighbour – a male with no known risk factors. After several months of living together and apparently engaging in sexual intercourse on a daily basis he also became anti-HIV positive.

Prostitutes thus may act as a reservoir for HIV transmission. It is known from several studies throughout major cities in the world that a proportion of prostitutes are infected with HIV. Despite the obvious potential risk of this group uncertainty exists since there are at present, excluding Africa, a relatively small number of AIDS cases among heterosexual males. Indeed it has even been suggested that males directly infected from prostitutes may have acquired HIV from infective semen remaining in the vagina from a previous client. Further it has been argued especially in Africa that treatment of sexually transmitted diseases caught as a result of contact with a prostitute may involve the use of non-sterile needles.

HIV has been isolated in menstrual blood and in cervical and vaginal secretions of antibody positive women. Like other sexually transmitted diseases the potential therefore exists for bidirectional (male to female, female to male) spread. It may be that transmission from female to male is less efficient than from male to female.

However, it can be seen that the potential for spread of HIV in the heterosexual community is a serious problem. It must be remembered that by far the largest category of AIDS patients consists of homosexual and bisexual men. In the UK at the end of December 1986 there were 610 AIDS patients of whom 538 are homosexual or bisexual. Other risk groups account for most of the remainder. Only 4 heterosexual, three women and one man, are presumed to have been infected in this country.

A further account of heterosexual spread is discussed below in cases associated with central Africa.

(6) CHILDHOOD AIDS

Children in the following categories are considered 'at risk' of acquiring HIV infection:

(1) Children born to HIV-antibody-positive mothers
(2) Children born to intravenous drug abusers or children who themselves abuse drugs intravenously
(3) Haemophiliacs and children born to haemophiliacs
(4) Children who are nationals of or who lived in Africa, Middle East, USA or the Caribbean
(5) Children from the above countries who have received blood transfusions especially in the neonatal period.

Reports of AIDS or a related syndrome in infants born to parents at risk from AIDS suggest that the virus is either passed from mother to child by the transplacental route or passage of the virus may occur via the mother's milk. Some researchers even feel that the virus inserts its genetic material into the germ cells of the host, and this allows transmission of the virus from generation to generation. But this theory still requires confirmation. As of 8 December 1986 in the United States 394 cases of infants with AIDS have been notified, with no marked male-to-female ratio. Of these children c. 79% have one or both parents who had AIDS or are members of high risk groups such as recipients of infected blood or blood products, intravenous drug abusers, bisexual men and haemophiliacs (see Table 1.5). The disease in children differs from that in adults in that only about half of the cases to date have fully-expressed AIDS, the remainder have a milder condition – the AIDS-related complex.

AIDS-related Kaposi's sarcoma in children, so far, is also rare. The incubation period is usually shorter and two clinical syndromes rarely seen in adult AIDS are common:

(a) Chronic swelling of the parotid salivary glands
(b) A rare chest infection called lymphocytic interstitial pneumonitis.

Perinatal transmission of AIDS is supported by:

(a) The early onset of illness in some of the infants.
(b) In many of the cases the patient's mother was in one of the high risk groups for developing AIDS.

In the United States recently, an infant of a male haemophiliac has developed AIDS along with the infant's mother. It was thought in this case that the AIDS agent was transmitted from male to female during normal heterosexual relations. The AIDS agent was then transmitted from mother to baby probably via the placenta (*in utero*) or during the process of birth. It is also possible that the AIDS agent was transferred after birth by breast milk or by maternal or paternal close contact with the baby.

In early July 1985 a baby in Sydney, Australia, became the world's first recorded victim to contract AIDS from his mother after being breast-fed. It is thought the mother had received the AIDS agent in a previous blood transfusion.

Transmission of HIV *in utero* has been observed as early as the 15th week of gestation; the risk of transmission is not precisely known but may occur in 50% or more of pregnancies in anti-HIV positive mothers.

Clinical features of childhood AIDS:
● Repeated infections especially diarrhoea, thrush, ear and upper respiratory tract
● Generalized swollen lymph glands
● Failure to thrive
● Delaying reaching developmental milestones
   See Appendix 5 for the Case Definition of AIDS in children.

(7) CASES ASSOCIATED WITH CENTRAL AFRICA

The AIDS virus has a very strong hold in parts of the African population. A 'concealed catastrophe' is going on in Africa.

Table 2.2   AIDS in Belgium and France: the African connection

Country	Total number of adult AIDS cases	African cases
Belgium	169	101
France	1 022	78

Data at 30 September 1986

AIDS appears to be occurring commonly in Zaire, Zambia, Uganda, Rwanda and other equatorial African countries. Among the cases of AIDS in Belgium and France there is a relatively large group which have links with Zaire (formerly the Belgian Congo), or with other central African countries (Figure 2.1 and Table 2.2).

The AIDS virus seems likely to have originated in central Africa since serum samples from the early 1970s show a high incidence of antibodies to the AIDS virus. No serum samples stored in the United States prior to 1978 have been shown to be antibody positive.

It is now apparent that an outbreak of AIDS has occurred in the western part of Zaire. In this outbreak however the risk groups have not been defined.

The presence of AIDS in central Africa is of considerable interest since it is in this area that Kaposi's sarcoma is endemic. The highest incidence in the world is found in Zaire where Kaposi's sarcoma accounts for almost 13% of all malignant cancers. It has been hypothesized that the high incidence of Kaposi's sarcoma in central Africa (particularly in Zaire) indicates that AIDS also originated in this region. The general lack of medical facilities and the presence of many other endemic infections could allow an immune deficiency disease not to be detected. Furthermore in a setting of high mortality in childhood, particularly from infectious diseases, cases of AIDS may go unrecognized. Severe protein-energy malnutrition in some children may predispose children to the AIDS agent or the reverse may be true. A recent report has shown that about 36% of children in Zaire have antibodies against the AIDS agent but this requires confirmation.

It has also been speculated that transmission of this disorder in rural Africa may be predominantly by homosexual contact although this is a taboo pastime in equatorial Africa as in Haiti and it is difficult to obtain information about the sexual life of Africans. Nevertheless the high degree of polygamy practised by the tribal

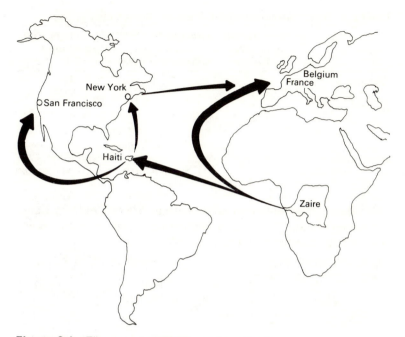

Figure 2.1   The spread of AIDS – an hypothesis

elders may encourage a homosexual phase in young males. Over the years about 14 000 Haitians have lived in Zaire and the hypothesis assumes that susceptible individuals took AIDS back to Haiti after their tour of duty (see Figure 2.1). Haiti is also a favoured holiday island for American homosexuals.

Recent evidence however suggests that heterosexual contact may be the main method of transmission among Africans. This is based on the following observations:

(a) The ratio of men to women in Africa with AIDS is one-to-one.

(b) The medical histories of patients with AIDS have shown that the important factor is the degree of exposure to the putative AIDS agent and not the type of sexual intercourse. There is also a high incidence of syphilis and gonorrhoea among the patients who develop AIDS.

(c) 'Clusters' of AIDS victims have occurred, many of whom have

Table 2.3   Sexual lifestyle and AIDS among African men

	Number who had regular contact with prostitutes	Average number of sexual partners per year	Percentage who had antibodies to AIDS virus
Patients ($n = 58$)	47 (81%)	32	87%
Controls ($n = 58$)	20 (34%)	3	14%

no known risk factor for AIDS but can be linked via sexual intercourse within the group.

(d) Spouses of patients with AIDS have a 75% risk of having antibodies against HIV. This indicates that at some time the spouse has been infected with the agent.

(e) About 80% of prostitutes in large cities in central Africa have antibodies to HIV. The repeated exposure to the AIDS agent through sexual intercourse has been blamed for this problem in equatorial Africa (see Table 2.3).

However, despite the compelling evidence of heterosexual transmission it is apparent that a high level of sexual activity is not the complete answer and as with AIDS in the United States and elsewhere co-factors such as sexually transmitted diseases and infectious tropical diseases (malaria, trypanosomiasis) may be involved. It is not thought that insect-borne transmission of the AIDS agent occurs. HIV cannot grow inside mosquito cells and the pattern of AIDS does not mirror that of other vector-borne diseases like malaria. More important factors include the use of unsterile needles and a history of sexually transmitted diseases in the past two years. However a recent article in the *South China Morning Post* has suggested that the AIDS agent might be transmitted by mosquitoes and 'other nasties such as bed bugs, lice and fleas . . . all voracious blood imbibers'. According to one report this has caused the sale of fly spray preparations in Hong Kong to rise at an explosive rate. So far there have been only three confirmed cases of AIDS in Hong Kong.

If the theory of heterosexual transmission of AIDS is correct this could have disastrous consequences. For example it would only need interaction between bisexual men and heterosexual women, or between homosexuals and prostitutes for widespread distribution of the AIDS agent. Many researchers however do not accept that AIDS will distribute itself so widely by heterosexual means. In this respect it has been proposed that AIDS is much more likely to be spread in Africa by dirty hypodermic syringes since it is quite common for queues of people undergoing vaccination to be injected with the same needle. Also in Africa injection is a popular way for drugs to be introduced into the body.

The emergence of AIDS from Africa could have come about due to population shifts from rural communities to cities. There would then be a greater chance of contact with foreign visitors who could carry the AIDS agent to new localities such as the United States. This is however speculation and the possibility has to be kept in mind that homosexual men could have introduced AIDS to Africa in a similar way as has been proposed in Haiti, that is by way of holidaying American homosexuals.

Finally it has been proposed that the AIDS epidemic was caused by the illicit activities of international blood brokers who bought cheap plasma from Central Africa and the Caribbean and sold it to American companies that manufacture factor VIII. Once the AIDS agent was introduced in this way it quickly spread, particularly in a promiscuous population with no natural resistance to the agent. This theory has been criticized on the grounds that the prevalence of AIDS in homosexuals is about seventy times that of haemophiliacs and AIDS was discovered in haemophiliacs only about a year after it was found in homosexuals. According to the originator of this theory, Dr Peter Jones: 'This takes the hooks out of the homosexual community, who are suffering a lot'. Transfusion banks in America deny involvement in blood brokerage but it is known that blood brokers operate everywhere in the world and buy and sell blood by telex. The Chief Medical Officer at the DHSS in England has recently stated that '. . . none of the plasma covered by current UK licences comes from areas where AIDS is known to be endemic'. Efforts are being made to make the United Kingdom self-sufficient in blood products and a redeveloped blood product laboratory will be opened in 1987 in Elstree, London. Dr Jones feels that government agencies should make public the source of blood products and at the same time submit blood to the best screening methods currently available.

At a recent conference a WHO official outlined the appalling situation in Africa. In parts of central Africa the virus is present in 10% of the population and 90% of prostitutes. A quarter of hospital patients have AIDS and a million Africans will die of AIDS in the next 10 years.

Most African governments except Uganda have chosen not to publicize the situation regarding AIDS. They have fears of reducing tourist revenue, or damaging foreign investment, or stimulating fear and racism in other countries. The facts of the incidence and prevalence of infections by HIV are therefore fragmentary and incomplete. By April 1986 blood tests had reliably confirmed the presence of HIV in at least 23 countries (see Figure 2.2). Data collected from city hospitals and large rural clinics have shown the following:

(1) 18% of blood donors in Kigali, Rwanda and 33% of men aged 30–35 in Lusaka and Zambia are carrying the AIDS virus.
(2) Among female prostitutes 27% in Kinshasa and 88% in Nairobi carry the AIDS virus.

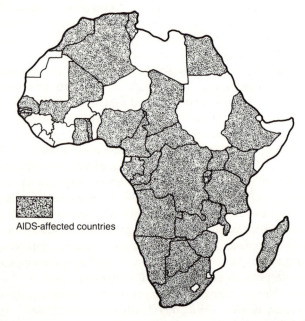

AIDS-affected countries

Figure 2.2   African countries known to be affected by AIDS (or HIV infection) as at November 1986. From Panos, *AIDS and the Third World*

(3) In 1980 in a Nairobi slum over 600 women who earn money through prostitution were tested for antibodies against the AIDS virus. None were positive. Recently they were tested again and now over 80% are HIV positive. Each woman averages about 1000 sexual partners a year (mostly truck drivers stopping for a 'tea-break' on their way from Mombasa). After some time many of the women will return to their villages, taking their children and HIV with them. New communities will then become infected.

(8) HAITIANS

The high prevalence of AIDS in Haitians living in Haiti or in those who have emigrated to the USA, Canada or France is not readily explained. In some of these patients homosexuality and drug abuse have not been obvious risk factors but in others they have. In addition, the question is raised regarding the localization of this disease to inhabitants of just this one Caribbean island. The incidence of AIDS principally in Haiti and the Americas – excluding the United States – is shown in Table 2.4. There has been a steady but not explosive growth of AIDS cases associated with Haiti.

One hypothesis is that Haiti could have been the actual source of the AIDS epidemic. However, in the opinion of experienced workers in Haiti, cases of AIDS were not seen on the island until 1979, one year after the current epidemic began. It therefore seems likely that AIDS in the United States pre-dates that in Haiti.

Exactly how the AIDS agent was transferred to Haiti is open to conjecture. A likely possibility is by homosexual contact with holidaying Americans for whom the island has been a fashionable resort. Relatively few Haitians, however, have admitted to homosexual activity due to cultural taboos against this practice. Nevertheless it is known that male homosexual prostitution occurs in this country. The male prostitutes are invariably heterosexual Haitian men, generally with families, who resort to this trade to supplement their otherwise meagre incomes.

It is therefore possible that homosexual contact between Haitians and American tourists could have introduced AIDS into Haiti. Having been established, the disease could then have spread rapidly by sexual contact in this small population.

Table 2.4 Acquired Immune Deficiency Syndrome in the Americas (excluding the United States) reported to WHO as of 14 November 1986

Country/area	Confirmed cases
Argentina	58
Bahamas	68
Barbados	4
Bermuda	42
Bolivia	1
Brazil	754
Canada	755
Chile	12
Colombia	5
Costa Rica	12
Cuba	1
Dominican Republic	62
Ecuador	7
El Salvador	2
French Guiana	31
Grenada	2
Guadeloupe	16
Guatemala	7
Haiti	501
Honduras	6
Jamaica	5
Martinique	6
Mexico	161
Panama	9
Peru	9
St Christopher & Nevis	1
Saint Lucia	10
St Vincent & the Grenadines	3
Surinam	2
Trinidad and Tobago	108
Uruguay	7
Venezuela	40
Total	2 707

Because of the uncertainty surrounding Haiti, and the recent evidence suggesting both heterosexual contact and exposure to contaminated needles, the CDC in March 1985 decide to drop Haitians as a separate risk group category in the published AIDS statistics. Haitian-born AIDS patients have now been placed into the

'Other/Unknown' group. The Haitians have complained of discrimination in America and a significant drop in tourism as a result of publicity surrounding AIDS.

CHAPTER 3

The cause of AIDS

At an early stage of the AIDS epidemic when the disease appeared to be confined to promiscuous homosexuals, it seemed possible that a toxic environmental agent might be implicated. A leading candidate was amyl nitrite (p. 55), a so-called street or recreational drug used to intensify sexual activity and for its general stimulant effects. Homosexuals use this drug and other nitrites such as isobutyl and butyl nitrite far more frequently than heterosexuals. The nitrites also act to relax the smooth muscle of the rectum and anal sphincter to facilitate anal intercourse.

Nitrite inhalants were implicated as a possible cause of AIDS for the following reasons.

(1) Nitrites are known mutagens and may have a role in the aetiology of Kaposi's sarcoma.
(2) Nitrites were thought to be immunotoxic and produce immune deficiency.
(3) On epidemiological grounds since the use of nitrite inhalants has been rare outside homosexual populations.

Some studies had suggested a positive connection between nitrite abuse and the risk of AIDS. However the results of case-controlled studies have indicated that nitrites are no longer regarded as a major factor in the cause of AIDS. Furthermore the nitrites have been shown to be non-immunotoxic in animals. However their role as a co-factor in this syndrome has not been ruled out.

A second hypothesis suggested that the basic immune defect in AIDS results from 'antigenic overload'. This is based on the findings that among homosexuals receptive (rather than insertive) anal intercourse represented a significant risk factor. Animal studies have indicated that sperm has an immunosuppressive effect. It was therefore suggested that homosexuals practising predominantly receptive anal intercourse are repeatedly exposed to sperm which induces immunosuppression. This, taken with the effects of the multiple infections that homosexuals suffer, was thought to result in a serious disruption of the immune system. However there are several weaknesses to this theory:

(1) It does not explain what causes the immune deficiency to become irreversible.
(2) It does not provide for the fact that AIDS is also a bloodborne disease.
(3) It does not explain why AIDS has occurred only recently.

Overwhelming evidence has accumulated in the last 1–2 years that suggests that AIDS is caused by a specific transmissible agent. The evidence for an infective cause of AIDS is supported by:

(1) The epidemic nature of the disease with the exponential rise.
(2) The pattern of patient groups at risk suggesting transmission by sexual, transplacental, perinatal or blood-to-blood contact.
(3) The geographical clustering of most cases.
(4) Direct evidence of case-to-case contact.

From the outset the causative agent for AIDS was thought to be a virus since:

(1) Viruses have been clearly demonstrated to be capable of causing immune deficiencies in man and animals, e.g. cytomegalovirus.
(2) In addition viruses are capable of inducing transformation and neoplasms in cell cultures (Epstein–Barr virus) and in animals (retroviruses) and probably in man (Epstein–Barr virus, retrovirus). This type of virus is called oncogenic since they can induce malignant transformation of normal cells.

A detailed discussion of the structure of viruses and viral diseases can be found in Appendix 6.

The balance of evidence strongly suggests that the causative agent of AIDS is a novel retrovirus which has been placed in the group Human T-cell Leukaemia Viruses. Since there are already two types of Human T-cell Leukaemia Virus the new virus implicated in AIDS was called Human T-cell Leukaemia Virus type III. More recently this virus was renamed as Human T-cell Lymphotropic Virus type III or HTLV-III since it does not cause leukaemia. In 1986 on the recommendation of the International Committee on the Taxonomy of viruses the virus identified as the causative agent of AIDS was renamed as the human immunodeficiency virus (HIV).

In 1986 a second virus HIV-2 was isolated in West Africa by two groups; one isolated it from AIDS patients and the other from healthy prostitutes. It is not clear whether these are the same or represent pathogenic variants.

The search for the AIDS agent has, however, been complicated by several problems:

(1) AIDS patients have often had prior exposure to multiple infections by sexually transmitted agents making it difficult to distinguish between the causative agent and the opportunists or passengers. For instance, almost all homosexual AIDS patients show evidence of infection with several viruses such as Epstein–Barr virus (EBV), cytomegalovirus (CMV), herpes virus types I and II, hepatitis B virus.

(2) Because of the derangement of the immune system in AIDS patients, potentially valuable serological techniques for identifying the infecting organisms may be ineffective because of the patient's acquired inability to form antibodies.

The AIDS agent itself could fall into one of two categories:

(1) A truly new agent.
(2) A familiar agent modified by mutation or some other co-factor to enable a new form of lethal expression.

A range of viruses had been considered possible causative agents for AIDS. These are:

(1) Hepatitis B virus
(2) Cytomegalovirus (CMV)
(3) Epstein–Barr virus (EBV)
(4) Retroviruses – Human T-cell Leukaemia viruses (HTLV)

For the sake of completeness the role of each of these viruses in the aetiology of AIDS is reviewed. Appendix 6 also provides useful background reading on viruses.

(1) HEPATITIS B VIRUS

The various hepatitis viruses (A, B, non A, non B), are so-called because they cause a liver infection first which usually presents as jaundice and general malaise. Hepatitis A or infectious hepatitis is caused by hepatitis A virus. It is commonly seen in epidemics and transmission of the virus is by the faecal–oral route. The disease is usually mild and self-limiting.

Hepatitis B or serum hepatitis is caused by hepatitis B virus. It is usually transmitted by injection of infected blood, or blood derivatives or by use of contaminated needles, lancets or other instruments. The disease is usually more severe than infectious hepatitis.

Since AIDS appeared in recipients of blood and blood products and in intravenous drug users, it was proposed that hepatitis B virus was the cause of AIDS. An alternative suggestion is that the virus may harbour the causative agent. This arises from the known ability of one surface particle on the virus, an antigen, to contain within itself a piece of genetic material quite separate and chemically different from the genetic material inside the virus. This so-called delta agent can also cause liver disease, independently of the virus, and may be even more serious than that caused by the virus itself. It had been speculated, therefore, that the delta agent or another separate piece of genetic material in the hepatitis B virus could be the cause of AIDS.

Evidence that hepatitis B virus may be implicated in AIDS has arisen from the following observations:

(a) Hepatitis B was an obvious candidate for the AIDS agent on the basis of similarities in the epidemiology of both infections:

   (i) About 90% of hepatitis B cases fall into one of three risk groups – homosexuals, intravenous drug users and haemophiliacs – since the virus is transmitted by blood and semen.

   (ii) Alone amongst the proposed viral agents hepatitis B virus infection spreads in a pattern very like that so far seen in AIDS, i.e. exponential growth rate with one individual infecting many others.

(b) About four-fifths of patients with AIDS have some serological marker (antibodies against hepatitis B virus) of past or current infection with hepatitis B virus.

However some observations do not support an association of hepatitis B virus with AIDS. These are:

(a) An increasingly large number of patients with AIDS have shown no evidence of hepatitis B infection.

(b) AIDS has not been recognized in other areas of the world where infection with hepatitis B is endemic and advanced medical care is available to diagnose AIDS, for example the Far East.

(c) Hepatitis B virus vaccine confers no protection against the development of AIDS when given to sexually active homosexuals.

On balance the evidence is more in favour of the hepatitis B virus acting as a passenger in AIDS rather than it being the causative agent.

Recently there has also been concern that the vaccine used to provide protection against hepatitis B may be contaminated with the AIDS agent. Hepatitis B vaccine (H-B-Vax) is prepared from the plasma of human carriers of the disease, often homosexuals. In the United Kingdom, people at high risk of contracting hepatitis B should be vaccinated. These include health care personnel in regular contact with blood or needles, or with patients in mental institutions; and patients who regularly receive blood products or blood transfusions. Failure to vaccinate these people may place them at unnecessary risk. Several researchers have demonstrated that there is no increased risk of AIDS in people who are vaccinated with H-B-Vax. Also it has been clearly shown that the AIDS agent (HIV) is killed by the purification processes used in H-B-Vax production. A further interesting parallel between the hepatitis B virus and the AIDS virus is the similarity in the route of transmission. It is now thought in homosexual men that, apart from contamination of partners with blood from lacerations in the rectum of the passive partner or cuts on the penis of the active partner, contaminated semen or saliva deposited in the rectum during anal intercourse or anal contact might be alternative modes of transmission.

Certainly it is well known that in Western countries more than 50% of homosexual men acquire hepatitis B within 2–3 years of indulgence in anal intercourse. It is widely accepted that the transmission of hepatitis B in homosexual men is through contact with infected blood or semen during anal intercourse.

(2) CYTOMEGALOVIRUS

Cytomegalovirus (CMV) is a large DNA virus and a member of the herpes family of viruses and is endemic throughout the world. Although cytomegalovirus infection is often asymptomatic or produces a mild glandular fever-like illness, the virus can cause eye infections and hepatitis. At various stages during infection the virus can be present in saliva, blood, semen, cervical secretions, urine and lymphocytes. Once cytomegalovirus infection is acquired the virus stays dormant indefinitely in body cells. Periodically it re-emerges from the latent state. This reactivation is known to occur when the immune status of the infected person is chronically depressed e.g. after cancer or chemotherapy or in the immunocompromised.

Several factors have suggested to some investigators that cytomegalovirus has an aetiological role in AIDS:

(a) Infection with cytomegalovirus is very common among homosexual men. In the United States 25–50% of heterosexual persons show evidence of previous or current infection with cytomegalovirus and greater than 90% of homosexuals and bisexuals. The high infection rate in these groups is probably the result of frequent sexual contact with CMV positive individuals. The status of IV drug users, haemophiliacs and Haitians with respect to CMV infection is less well studied, but these groups should reasonably be expected to have high infection rates as well.

(b) Cytomegalovirus can cause immune suppression either due to systemic infection or perhaps due to infection at unusual sites, e.g. via semen. For example CMV activates suppressor T-cells resulting in a reduction in the ratio of T-helper cells to T-suppressor cells to produce adverse effects on the immune system.

(c) Cytomegalovirus is transmitted transplacentally, by sexual contact (transfer in semen and excreta) or by blood transfusion from acutely infected individuals or from individuals with reactivated disease.

(d) Cytomegalovirus DNA has been found in Kaposi's sarcoma tumour cells and may play a role in the expression or transformation process resulting in the development of clinical Kaposi's sarcoma.

Although a case for CMV association with AIDS has been put forward it seems likely that CMV is probably reactivated as a result of immunosuppression or is acquired as an opportunistic infection and is therefore not directly involved in the aetiology of AIDS.

(3) EPSTEIN–BARR VIRUS

Epstein–Barr virus (EBV), like CMV, is a member of the herpes family of viruses and has an affinity for lymphoid cells. It is the most common cause of glandular fever (infectious mononucleosis) in young people. It is widely distributed throughout the world and after infection an individual usually harbours the virus in a dormant state for life.

Reasons for considering Epstein–Barr virus in the aetiology of AIDS include:

(a) The virus is closely associated with certain malignancies, especially Burkitt's lymphoma which is one of the cancers occurring in AIDS (see later). In Burkitt's lymphoma the Epstein–Barr virus induces malignancies within the B-lymphocytes.

(b) Epstein–Barr virus has known immune effects e.g. T-lymphocyte helper/suppressor ratios are altered during acute attacks.

The pronounced preference of the Epstein–Barr virus for the B-cell (antibody-producing) component of the immune system suggests that the virus is not solely responsible for the predominant T-cell defect in AIDS. In addition the occurrence of Burkitt's lymphoma in immunosuppressed transplant patients as well as in AIDS patients indicates that the virus is another opportunist rather than the primary cause of AIDS. It appears that EBV and CMV are opportunist pathogens that become established after immunosuppression has occurred.

(4) RETROVIRUSES

A retrovirus is an RNA virus able to make DNA which may then be inserted into the host cell DNA or genetic machinery. The virus is then able to use the host cell's replicative machinery to reproduce itself as well as make various substances that have been shown to cause transformation of host cells into malignant cells. The ability of retroviruses to make DNA from RNA is the result of the presence of an enzyme called reverse transcriptase. Transcription describes the formation of RNA from DNA. Reverse transcription therefore results in the formation of DNA from RNA. Retroviruses, RNA tumour viruses, were considered among the more likely AIDS agent candidates because:

(a) Some retroviruses have a specificity for lymphocytes.
(b) The viruses are blood-borne.
(c) Some of the retroviruses can cause immunodeficiency in animals: e.g. the feline leukaemia virus causes immunosuppression in cats (Feline–AIDS). A spontaneous outbreak of a disease in monkeys (Simian AIDS or 'SAIDS') which had similarities to AIDS was caused by a retrovirus.
(d) In man a group of retroviruses known as human T-cell leukaemia virus (HTLV) have been associated with certain malignancies of T-lymphocytes and can produce T-cell over-production leading to leukaemia.

The first two human T-cell leukaemia viruses to be characterized were:

(a) Human T-Cell Leukaemia Virus-1 (HTLV-I)
    This is associated with adult T-cell leukaemia which is par-
    ticularly prevalent in south west Japan, the Caribbean, regions
    of South America and Africa. The virus, HTLV-I, causes T-
    cells to proliferate uncontrollably and transforms T-cells into
    tumour cells. About 1% of Japanese are HTLV-I carriers and
    about 30% of people living in the endemic area have antibodies
    to HTLV-I but only about 0.05% of them develop adult T-cell
    leukaemia. It may be that other factors such as the host immune
    response, virus dose or route of infection are important in disease
    manifestation.
        Japanese researchers have shown that normal human lym-
    phocytes can be transformed into cancerous lymphocytes by
    culturing them with leukaemic cells from a patient with adult T-
    cell leukaemia.

It is thought that Asian Old World monkeys may have 'carried' the virus to these distinct geographical areas since these primates succumb to a leukaemia very similar to adult T-cell leukaemia. Further it is thought that some individuals of African descent may have increased susceptibility to infection with both HTLV-I and HTLV-III.

(b) Human T-cell Leukaemia Virus-2 (HTLV-II)

This is a much rarer HTLV variant which has been isolated from only a few patients with hairy cell leukaemia – a very rare leukaemia. HTLV-II appears at present, though, not to be associated with any specific disease. Further studies are required to determine its worldwide distribution.

A possible association with AIDS was investigated for both viruses on the basis of their affinity for T-helper cells and their prevalence in Africa and Haiti among other areas.

However reliable evidence of infection with HTLV-I and HTLV-II was found to be limited to only a small proportion of AIDS patients. Human T-cell leukaemia virus isolates were identified in only 10% of patients. 25% of cases had antibodies against HTLV. Most workers have concluded that HTLV-I and HTLV-II, if present, are passengers in AIDS and not the causative agent.

HUMAN IMMUNODEFICIENCY VIRUS (HIV), formerly called human T-cell lymphotropic virus III (HTLV-III), lymphadenopathy-associated virus (LAV)

Recently a third member of the family of Human T-cell Leukaemia Viruses has been discovered and is thought to be the putative or causative agent of AIDS and is more properly called the human immunodeficiency virus (HIV). The evidence for this is based on the following observations:

(1) HIV has been isolated from blood, semen, saliva and tears of patients with AIDS.

(2) HIV has been isolated in a high percentage of:
   (a) ● AIDS cases
       ● AIDS cases with Kaposi's sarcoma

- AIDS cases with opportunistic infection
- Children with AIDS
- Mothers of such children
- Clinically normal homosexual blood donors
- Pre-AIDS patients

The detection rate of HIV isolates is probably lower than the true incidence since it may be more difficult to detect virus-infected T-cells in patients with advanced AIDS because the susceptible cell population is so severely depleted in these patients.

(b) In patients with the AIDS prodrome (persistent generalized lymphadenopathy (PGL), fever, malaise and weight loss are thought to be a sign of incipient AIDS).

(c) Symptomless homosexuals.

No normal control donors outside the high risk groups showed any evidence of HIV.

(3) Antibodies to HIV have been detected in:
- AIDS patients
- PGL patients
- Symptomatic homosexuals
- Contacts of AIDS or PGL patients
- Homosexuals at risk
- Haemophiliacs who have received pooled clotting factors
- Intravenous drug abusers.

The excellent study that produced the list above also demonstrated that no antibody was present for over one thousand unselected control blood donors.

(4) HIV is toxic *in vitro* to helper T-cells. Low helper T-cell counts are characteristic of the immunological defect found in AIDS patients.

HIV shows marked similarities to a retrovirus previously isolated in France, called the lymphadenopathy-associated virus (LAV). The lymphadenopathy-associated virus was first identified by Professor Luc Montagnier and his team at the Pasteur Institute in Paris in May 1983 when they isolated the virus from a homosexual man with lymphadenopathy. This was followed almost one year later by the identification of HTLV-III by Dr Robert Gallo at the National Cancer Institute in Bethesda, Maryland, USA, in May 1984. To make matters more complicated a third group of researchers headed by Dr Levy from San Francisco have isolated this virus but refer to it as AIDS-related virus (ARV). It seems however that Gallo and Montagnier are the front runners in this particular race and, no doubt, either or both of these researchers are in line for a Nobel Prize, let alone any commercial implications of their discovery. The similarities between LAV and HTLV-III and ARV are as follows:

(1) HTLV-III, LAV and ARV demonstrate selective infection of T-helper cells.

(2) Isolates of HTLV-III, lymphadenopathy-associated virus and ARV have also been identified in AIDS patients.

(3) HTLV-III, LAV and ARV antibodies have been detected with similar frequency in various groups:
   (a) AIDS patients
   (b) Patients with AIDS prodrome
   (c) Symptom-free homosexuals at risk
   (d) Normal donors from Central Africa

(4) HTLV-III, LAV and ARV have RNA as their genetic material.

(5) All three viruses appear very similar under the electron microscope.

(6) Assay tests indicate that the three viruses are indistinguishable.

(7) The genetic codes ('fingerprints') are essentially indistinguishable for the three viruses.

HTLV-III, LAV and ARV are therefore now thought to be one and the same virus and this has been renamed human immunodeficiency virus HIV.

But research is moving so quickly in this area that it may be that the three viruses, although bearing many similarities, belong to different taxonomic groups. Also recently, it has been argued that since HTLV-I and HTLV-II do not destroy lymphocytes but HTLV-III clearly does that the causative virus in AIDS does not belong in the same class. HTLV-I and HTLV-II cause T-cell proliferation and hence leukaemia; HIV causes T-helper cell death and immune deficiency.

However for the purpose of simplicity the AIDS virus will be referred to as HIV throughout this text. The evidence that HIV is the causative agent for AIDS is compelling:

(1) The frequency of virus isolation from AIDS and related disorders is relatively high.

(2) Isolation has been achieved in a range of high risk patient groups including Africans and children.

(3) The level of antibody formation to HIV is high in AIDS and in the AIDS prodrome.

(4) There is direct evidence for sexual, blood-borne and vertical transmission (i.e. from mother to child).

(5) There is clear specificity for T-helper cells, the portion of the immune system most commonly defective in AIDS.

(6) HIV antibodies have not been detected in patients whose immune system has been disrupted due to other factors such as immunosuppressive drugs, lymphomas, congenital immune deficiencies etc. This suggests that HIV is involved in the cause of the immune deficiency in AIDS rather than just a consequence of it.

Origins of HIV

The origins of the human immunodeficiency virus are not totally clear. It has been suggested, but not confirmed, that the virus has been man-made in the Soviet Union or United States as a weapon of biological warfare. There is a good deal of support for the theory that HIV first emerged from central Africa although the African governments steadfastly contest this theory. Recent research has shown that a very similar virus called Simian T-cell lymphotropic virus type III (STLV-III) is present in the Asian and African macaque monkey. Antibodies to the AIDS virus strongly cross-react with STLV-III.

Theories concerning the source and evolution of HIV are therefore only provisional and it is an area of intensive research since such

information would also prove valuable to the search for a vaccine
against the virus.

Pathogenesis of HIV infection

Human immunodeficiency virus (HIV) infects only specific cells of
the immune system, the groups of T-lymphocytes known as T-helper
cells. The underlying defect in AIDS may, therefore, be a direct result
of too few T-helper cells to produce a normal immune response (see
Appendix 4).

(1) A depletion in T-helper cells would cause an impaired B-cell
    antibody response. T-helper cells essentially give B-cells 'per-
    mission' to produce antibodies and direct B-cells in exactly which
    antibody to produce to meet a specific antigen. T-cells also
    increase the rate of B-cell production.

(2) A depletion in T-helper cells would cause a reduction in the
    response of cytotoxic T-cells and suppressor T-cells to antigen.

(3) A depletion in T-helper cells would cause a decrease in the
    production of substances known as lymphokines which activate
    the various white blood cells including lymphocytes. For
    instance, the lymphokine interleukin II binds to receptors on the
    surface of T-cells and stimulates them to grow and divide.

The severity of the underlying immunological dysfunction does,
however, suggest that the defect may be broader than simply T-cell
depletion. Possibly it is attributable in part to the relative excess of
T-suppressor cells. These lymphocytes determine when B-cells have
produced sufficient antibody to effectively eliminate an antigen and
then release specific lymphokines that suppress further antibody
production. Normally as we have seen previously there are twice as
many helper cells as suppressor cells; in AIDS this ratio is reversed,
due to a loss of helper cells (see Appendix 4).

Thus an hypothesis for the pathogenetic process involves the
following steps:

(1) *Infection*
    The virus (HIV) infects a T-lymphocyte helper cell possibly only

of a particular subset of T-helper cells. This step may be clinically inapparent.

(2) *T-cell activation*
Evidence suggests that the virus replicates fastest when the T-cell is in an activated state. This occurs when it is stimulated by an antigen. The T-cell then rapidly divides to produce a clone of genetically identical cells which are able to combat the invader or antigen. In AIDS certain antigenic co-factors may cause the T-cell to become activated. Possible co-factors are previous viral infection, multiple infections by sexually transmitted diseases, exposure to the antigenic components of semen, frequent infusions of blood products etc.

(3) *Replication*
In the activated T-helper cell, the virus (HIV) is able to replicate and consequently spread to a larger portion of T-helper cells. Several cell cycles may be needed before T-cell depletion through lysis or some other mechanism of elimination leads to clinical immunodeficiency. This may account for the variable and some-times long latent period before clinical symptoms are manifest. It also indicates that infection with HIV can be associated with a variety of outcomes (Figure 3.1):

  (a) Asymptomatic carriers
  (b) Persistent generalized lymphadenopathy (PGL)
  (c) Symptomatic lymphadenopathy or AIDS-related complex (ARC)
  (d) AIDS

The answer to the question concerning what triggered HIV to be transformed to its present sinister character is still not known.

CO-FACTORS INVOLVED IN HIV INFECTION

Whether infection with the viral agent is sufficient alone to cause the Acquired Immune Deficiency Syndrome remains to be seen; co-factors that may be involved in this process include:

(1) Genetic susceptibility
(2) Immunosuppression by semen

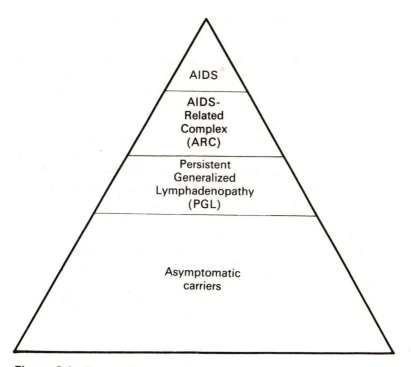

Figure 3.1 The spectrum of HIV infection

(3) Immunosuppression by cytomegalovirus
(4) Recreational drug use

(1) Genetic susceptibility

As yet the extent to which susceptibility to HIV infection is determined by individual genetic make-up is not known. It is apparent that while many individuals may be exposed to the AIDS agent, as in the case of haemophiliacs using factor VIII concentrate, only a few will develop the illness. The genetic constitution as well as other factors, such as age of the individual when infected, may well explain this discrepancy.

(2) Immunosuppression by semen

Homosexual AIDS patients are repeatedly exposed not only to viruses but also to semen which may enter the blood stream through lacerated rectal tissue during rectal intercourse. The rectum is designed to withdraw water from faecal matter and will readily absorb components of semen. By comparison the wall of the vagina is thicker and less likely to tear during sexual intercourse and is also relatively impermeable to semen. Sperm and other chemical substances are also inactivated by vaginal secretions.

Semen from another person is treated by the body as a foreign substance, an antigen, which triggers the production of antibodies against it. Such antibodies have, however, been shown to act as auto-antibodies; that is their action is directed not just against foreign semen but also against the body's own cells and in particular the T-lymphocytes. The overall effect is a suppression of the immune response. So far this has only been positively seen in mice. Nevertheless it is possible that repeated exposure to semen produces a background of immune suppression which may trigger expression of the AIDS virus.

(3) Immunosuppression by cytomegalovirus

Cytomegalovirus (CMV) infection appears to be common in all AIDS risk groups and in AIDS patients and is found in the saliva, urine and semen. As with some other viral infections CMV infection can produce immunosuppressive effects by activating T-suppressor cells. Although the immune deficiency tends to be transient it may still add to the host's susceptibility to AIDS particularly if it augments the possible immune dysfunction caused by semen. Cytomegalovirus like EBV, herpes viruses and HIV is a latent infection and in common with this group of viruses is able to remain dormant in the body for many years.

(4) Recreational drugs

The use of nitrite inhalants or 'poppers' which contain either amyl or butyl nitrite is one of the well-known differences between homo-sexuals and heterosexuals; homosexuals use these recreational drugs more frequently than heterosexuals.

Amyl nitrite was originally used to help overcome the chest pain of angina by its vasodilatory action on the coronary blood vessels of the heart.

In the United Kingdom amyl nitrite has now been largely replaced by other drugs although it is still available from chemists without prescription. In the United States, however, amyl nitrite was freely available but now can be sold only with a prescription. As a result a closely related chemical, butyl nitrite (marketed as an odourizer) is also used as a recreational drug. Inhaling nitrites produces a pleasant physical effect with a brief intensification of sexual sensi-tivity. They also cause relaxation of the smooth muscle of the rectum and anal sphincter thus facilitating anal intercourse.

Exactly why homosexuals should use these agents to a greater degree than heterosexual men is unclear, and this suggested initially that there might be an association with AIDS. However, surveys of homosexual AIDS patients revealed an increasing number of cases who had never used nitrite inhalants. In addition, the immuno-suppressive effect that these drugs were shown to cause in mice could not be substantiated in man.

'Poppers' are not thought to entail any significant risk in associ-ation with AIDS. Neither has a statistical relationship been dis-covered between AIDS and the use of other drugs such as amphetamines, barbiturates, heroin, cocaine, glue, cannabis or LSD.

Poppers may help to increase the amount of high risk sex that a person has and therefore increase the likelihood of HIV infection. There is also the possibility that nitrites may enhance the trans-mission of viruses by causing capillary vasodilation in the rectal mucosa.

CHAPTER 4

Transmission of the AIDS virus

On the basis of the risk groups which have been identified with AIDS there is evidence to suggest that the AIDS virus is transmitted:

(1) By sexual contact – homosexual and heterosexual
(2) By parenteral transfer in blood or blood products
(3) By shared needles and syringes – intravenous drug users
(4) By transplacental and perinatal transfer from mother to child

HIV has been isolated from lymphocytes in peripheral blood, bone marrow cells, spinal fluid and brain tissue, lymph nodes, cell free plasma, saliva, semen and tears. Exposure to any of these body fluids, if contaminated, represents a risk. However the risk of infection depends heavily on the route of exposure.

There is currently no evidence of the spread of the AIDS virus by casual social contact or shaking hands; the virus is not transmissible in ordinary daily activities. The virus cannot be caught by touching objects used by an infected person: cups, cutlery, clothes, towels, toilet seats and door knobs. HIV is a very fragile virus and does not tolerate heat; 60°C kills the virus. Many disinfectants including household bleach destroy the virus.

(1) SEXUAL CONTACT

Sexual intercourse between males or a male and female transfers the AIDS virus in the semen. It appears at present, that there is only a low risk of transmission from an infected woman to a man. Meanwhile Britain's largest artificial insemination organization, the British Pregnancy Advisory Service, and some American organizations have started to screen all semen donors for the presence of HIV antibodies. To date there have been 4 cases of AIDS reported to have occurred following artificial insemination.

Among homosexuals the activity which carries the highest risk of infection with the AIDS virus is receptive anal intercourse. Insertive anal intercourse by comparison is thought to carry less risk of AIDS and may correspond to the low rate of AIDS transmission from women to men by sexual intercourse.

Exposure to the partner's faeces during sexual activity may also predispose to HIV infection.

The combination of frequent receptive anal intercourse with many homosexual partners probably involves the greatest risk for HIV infection. Promiscuity among homosexuals was highlighted at an early stage of the AIDS epidemic as a significant risk factor. One report stated that AIDS patients on average had 62 partners per year against 25 partners per year for healthy controls. Some AIDS cases have had more than 100 sexual partners a year and one individual claimed an average of 90 partners a month during the year before diagnosis (a staggering 1080 partners a year). The early cases tended to have more partners but recently patients with AIDS appear to be not so promiscuous. It may be that the AIDS virus has spread widely through the gay community as a result of a minority of highly promiscuous individuals.

In the United Kingdom and other European countries multiple sexual partners are thought not to be so prevalent. The law in the United Kingdom for instance, makes homosexual group sex and sex in public places illegal so the opportunities for promiscuity are relatively limited. This is in marked contrast to the United States where special facilities exist for homosexuals such as backrooms, gay bars, gay bath-houses etc. which encourage casual or anonymous sex. Recently in California in an attempt to control AIDS, homosexual bath-houses, bars and other facilities were closed. However these were allowed to re-open but with a ban on high risk sex acts such as anal sex, fellatio (oral sex), blood biting, sharing sex toys or needles etc.

There is some evidence now that the newly-diagnosed cases of AIDS in American homosexuals are more restrained in their sexual activities with as few as 2–4 partners a year. Since it is known that HIV is present in semen in infected individuals multiple sexual partners may only be a risk factor in as much as it increases the likelihood of contact with an infected individual and increases the frequency of exposure. However, other factors such as repeated exposure to antigenic components in the semen and viral infection may also be involved and exacerbate the primary infection.

Analyses of risks associated with different sexual activities of AIDS patients and controls have given equivocal results. In one study, AIDS patients were significantly more likely than controls to have histories of 'fisting' or inserting a fist or forearm into a partner's rectum, and of 'rimming' or inserting their tongue into a partner's anus. The relative risk of other commonly conducted sexual practices such as fellatio, and 'water sports' or micturating onto a partner is not clear but they are best avoided.

The overall impact of multiple sexual partners, however, has been to amplify the transmission of the AIDS agent. Sexual activity in a setting of casual sex with multiple sometimes anonymous partners had led to the spread of AIDS with epidemic proportions.

There is also a body of opinion that suggests that AIDS is a classic blood-borne viral disease, rather like hepatitis B. In both diseases homosexual men are at increased risk because they partake in anal intercourse. The wall of the rectum is relatively thin and the skin of the penis is fragile. Minor injuries would allow small amounts of blood and hence virus to be passed from one sexual partner to another. This is an interesting theory and requires further research but it is thought that the rectal wall is easier to penetrate by micro-organisms than the thicker vaginal wall.

(2) PARENTERAL TRANSFER

There is ample evidence that blood, blood products or factor VIII concentrate obtained from AIDS patients carries the causative agent. However, for transmission to occur it appears that the infected blood must be introduced directly into the blood stream of the recipient. Contaminated blood falling on the skin or on food is probably not sufficient to cause subsequent infection.

Prevention of transfusion-associated HIV infection depends on three precautions:

(a) Efficient methods of screening of donors through health education so that persons at high risk are either dissuaded from attending the donor session or exclude themselves at the centre.

(b) The availability of a sensitive and reliable test for the presence of HIV.

(c) The use of a method of inactivating HIV that increases the safety factor without significantly destroying the blood product.

For further details see the section on haemophilia and blood transfusion patients in Chapter 2.

(3) PERINATALLY (VERTICAL TRANSMISSION)

Infants may acquire AIDS *in utero* or via their mother's milk, or via close contact after birth. For further details see the section on childhood AIDS in Chapter 2.

It is also known that the AIDS virus is found in cervical secretions and menstrual blood from infected women and this may account for the means of transfer of virus during vaginal intercourse. The virus would pass through any abrasion or break in the lining of the penis. It has even been suggested that uncircumcised males are at greater risk since the inner lining of the penis can represent about 50% of the surface area of the shaft when the penis is erect, thereby increasing the risk that the AIDS virus will be acquired through a skin break. Although unconfirmed this is an interesting observation since it is known that both genital herpes and syphilis are more common in uncircumcised men. Both of these diseases depend on a break or abrasion in the skin to gain entry into the body.

(4) SALIVARY TRANSFER

The existence of HIV in human saliva has recently been demonstrated. The virus has been isolated in individuals with the AIDS prodrome or from those who had had contact with AIDS patients. This raises the possibility that the putative AIDS agent could be passed on by kissing or in an airborne form from coughing and sneezing. The next step must, therefore, be to determine the infectious potential of salivary transfer. Researchers have to date failed to report how much of the virus is contained in the saliva. So far there is no epidemiological evidence to suggest that people have been infected by this route. There is, of course, overwhelming evidence that sexual and blood-to-blood transfer are more important.

As a precaution the Australian Dental Association has now recommended that dentists should wear gloves as a routine and masks and eye protection should be worn while treating 'high risk' subjects. It has recently been pointed out in the *British Dental Journal* that asking patients if they, their spouse or parent is gay, bisexual, a prostitute, or mainlining heroin is not the best way to build up a private practice. However, concern among dentists has been high and the British Dental Association reports 'voluminous' enquiries on the risks associated with AIDS.

Epidemiological evidence suggests that AIDS can be transmitted not only by patients with the disease but also by subjects who are well, or in a prodromal phase of the illness, who are acting as 'carriers' of the AIDS agent. Only by identification of all infectious individuals, whether symptomatic or not, can there be any hope of curbing the present epidemic and preventing a widespread outbreak in the population as a whole.

Early in 1985 in the United Kingdom there was much public and media concern regarding the possible transmission of AIDS through contact with infected saliva. The Fire Brigades Union among others advised its members not to offer mouth-to-mouth resuscitation to anyone they suspected of being homosexual. According to Gay Switchboard, an information service for homosexuals, men have been asked to leave some working men's clubs and public houses because they were suspected of being homosexual. The fear was that beer glasses could become tainted with the AIDS virus. Even Church leaders have questioned the British Government regarding the possibility of infection with AIDS virus by the use of the 'common cup' in Holy Communion services. The risk of transmission of the AIDS virus in such cases is reported to be negligible. Indeed the wine in the chalice would probably render the virus inactive.

Some recent research has further shown that salivary transmission is unlikely. Chimpanzee and human saliva completely inhibited the ability of HIV to infect human white blood cells. Further investigation revealed that saliva contains two inhibitory substances that inactivate the AIDS virus.

There is also much anecdotal evidence that saliva is an unlikely source of infection. One of these concerns a woman, who after being bitten in the finger by a man with AIDS, still shows no sign of infection 18 months later.

INCUBATION PERIOD OF THE AIDS VIRUS

The early pattern of slow growth in the United States epidemic suggested that a relatively long incubation period of several years was involved following infection with the AIDS agent. More specific evidence has defined a latent period of the disease from about 6 months to more than 6 years. The average incubation period is about 28 months.

This is based on the following observations:

(1) Cases of AIDS have occurred in which blood products were the only presumed exposure to the HIV. In these instances precise information could be obtained concerning the initial infection and subsequent clinical expression of the illness.

(2) Contact tracing revealed that an individual who had homosexual contact with an AIDS patient subsequently developed symptoms of the disease about 1 year after contact.

(3) A report of New York State prisoners who had been intravenous drug users but who developed AIDS months after their imprisonment. (A good deal of intravenous drug abuse is still found in prisons in the United States and the United Kingdom.)

CHAPTER 5

Infection with the AIDS virus

Following infection with HIV, antibodies to HIV usually appear within a period of about 8 weeks. This process, called seroconversion, may result in a transient non-specific glandular fever-type illness, but usually there are no symptoms. The acute phase of infection during which antibodies develop is followed by a chronic phase which may also be asymptomatic or it may be accompanied by illness. The symptomatic classification of chronic HIV infection is best divided into:

(1) Persistent Generalized Lymphadenopathy (PGL)
(2) AIDS-related complex (ARC)
(3) Fully expressed AIDS

TESTS FOR THE AIDS VIRUS

Introduction

There are currently three approaches to detecting HIV infection; listed in increasing order of difficulty these are

(a) Detection of HIV-specific antibodies produced by infected person's immune system
(b) Detection of viral antigens present in blood
(c) Detection of HIV by culturing it.

Two tests, both of type (a), are used in the current testing programme. One of these ELISA (see later) reacts to the presence of antibodies in the donor's blood, showing a more intense colour as larger quantities of the antibodies are present in serum. If the test is positive, usually two further ELISA tests are performed. If either is positive the blood is classified as repeatedly reactive. For final confirmation and to rule out any possible errors (see later) a second test called Western blot is then applied. The Western blot test also detects antibody but it gives more specific information about the particular antibodies produced against the many HIV antigens. It is more expensive but is less likely to give a false positive or false negative result (see later).

If the specimen is ELISA and Western blot positive the donor is regarded as infected with HIV and the donor is notified.

The most specific test for HIV infection is isolation of the virus; however HIV is difficult to isolate in cell culture and this remains impractical for large-scale use.

In February 1985 the United States Government's Food and Drug Administration (FDA) approved a commercial test for identifying blood that is contaminated with antibodies produced against the AIDS virus. Antibodies are produced as an immunological response against the virus but in the majority of cases the antibodies confer no protection against the underlying infection. The test (from Abbott Laboratories) is known as ELISA (Enzyme-Linked Immuno-Sorbent Assay) and detects only the antibodies that the donor has produced in response to infection from the AIDS virus. The ELISA test is performed in three stages (see Figure 5.1). In the first stage the AIDS virus is disrupted and particles (antigens) are attached to a plastic sheet. Human serum is added in the second stage. If the person has been previously infected with the virus, the serum will contain antibodies which will bind to the antigens attached to the plastic sheet. Unbound serum antibody is washed away and in the third stage an anti-antibody is added. The anti-antibody is usually made by injecting a goat with human antibody (immunoglobulin). The anti-human antibody from the goat is then labelled with an enzyme which produces a colour reaction when it reacts with a specific chemical. In the final stage labelled anti-antibody is added as a marker and excess anti-antibody is again washed away. If the human serum contains antibodies against the AIDS virus it will have bound to the AIDS virus on the plastic sheet. This in turn will have bound the labelled goat antibody. If when substrate is added a colour

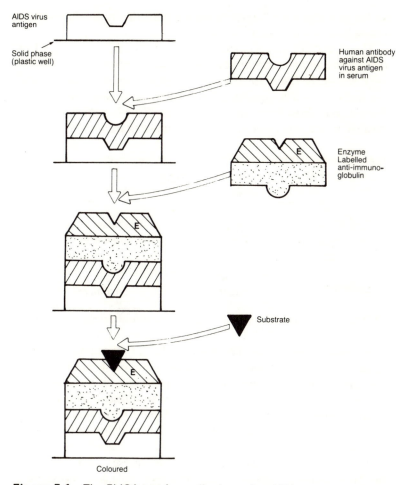

AIDS virus antigen

Solid phase (plastic well)

Human antibody against AIDS virus antigen in serum

Enzyme Labelled anti-immuno-globulin

Substrate

Coloured

Figure 5.1 The ELISA test for antibody against HIV

forms this means the person has at some time been infected with the AIDS virus. In the USA the ELISA test is likely to be the 'test of choice' for repeat testing of blood. The test provides no clue as to whether the virus is still present or whether it has been destroyed by the body. However recent studies have shown the presence of HIV virus in about 90% of homosexuals with a positive antibody test. It appears that once infected with the AIDS virus individuals remain so for many years at least. A person with the antibodies will not necessarily go on to develop AIDS.

The American Government's Public Health Service has ordered that all blood donations in the United States, about 1.5 million per year, should be tested for the presence of antibodies. Unfortunately the test-kit is not foolproof – it sometimes detects antibodies when further tests show there are none present. This is known as a false-positive result (see Table 5.1) and is thought to occur at a frequency

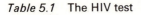

Table 5.1 The HIV test

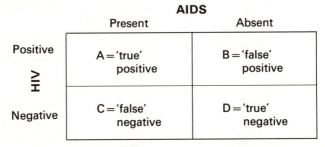

	AIDS	
	Present	Absent
HIV Positive	A = 'true' positive	B = 'false' positive
HIV Negative	C = 'false' negative	D = 'true' negative

of less than 1.0% of all tests. A false-positive test result may occur as a result of cross-reaction of antibodies produced as a result of infection with an antigenically related virus or it may be caused by non-specific test factors. Conversely the test-kit may not detect antibodies when further tests show they are present. This is known as a false-negative result (see Table 5.1) and there is a risk in this situation that blood donors with a positive antibody test would slip through the net.

There is therefore much criticism of the present test that it may not be accurate enough to be used on a wide scale, and British blood transfusion specialists have recently opposed introducing any test that gives a high rate of false-positives. Screening for antibody to HIV is already routine in the United States and West Germany and by October 1985 was available in the UK. Such screening may result in the loss of some donors and the attraction of high risk individuals wanting to know their antibody status.

In June 1985 the directors of the United Kingdom haemophilia reference centre expressed their concern about the safety of blood and unheated blood products. This group of doctors suggested that in certain patients such as those undergoing heart surgery or those receiving large quantities of blood or blood products the risk of HIV infection in such patients could be as high as one in 200 in some parts of Britain. They concluded that 'although testing for HIV antibodies will be expensive it should be implemented as soon as possible to protect recipients and to preserve public confidence in our blood transfusion services'. The Health Minister in the United Kingdom announced in October 1985 that routine testing for HIV antibodies was to be introduced at blood transfusion centres. Arrangements were also being made for counselling of blood donors later found to be truly positive for antibodies. All donated blood is now tested for HIV antibody and all factor VIII now supplied is heat-treated.

At least four other American pharmaceutical and biotechnology companies (Dupont, Electronucleonics, Litton and Travenol–Genentech Diagnostics) are competing for the highly lucrative test-kit market estimated to be worth about $80 million per year in the United States. Also the tests show only if the patient has been exposed to the virus, not when. The antibody test is not a test for AIDS since it cannot predict if the patient is still infected with the AIDS virus or has already successfully fought off an attack. The test therefore is probably of little use during the early stages of the infection when the body is producing antibody in response to the virus. This occurs in about the first few months after the virus has been 'caught'. It may also occur early on in some people with AIDS whose immune system is suppressed and therefore cannot mount an adequate immunological response to the invasion by the virus. It is thought that about 5% of those in whom the virus is present give a negative antibody test. A negative test result therefore does not necessarily mean a person is non-infectious.

In the UK both Wellcome and Organon Technika have antibody tests approved for use. One utilises ELISA whereas the other is based on a slightly different technique.

A recent analysis of over 15 000 plasma samples from random blood donors in the United States showed that 236 samples were consistently positive for antibodies to HIV. From this result it is clear that even though special screening of donors for AIDS had been in place before the samples were collected, individuals with HIV antibody were still donating blood. It was not possible to check if the seropositive donors were from the well defined 'risk group' for AIDS.

Haemophiliacs appear to develop antibodies and AIDS less frequently than homosexuals. It is thought that this may be because the virus was in part inactivated during the preparation of blood products. The 'weakened' virus may therefore be less likely to establish itself and cause AIDS in those haemophiliacs at risk.

For every haemophiliac who has received factor VIII concentrate and who has contracted AIDS there are at least 700 to 800 others receiving concentrates from the same blood lots who have not contracted the syndrome. Some of these however may be antibody-positive but asymptomatic. Obviously there are significant but as yet unknown factors other than the clotting factor preparation which determine whether a patient receiving factor VIII will contract AIDS. Recently in Scotland a contaminated batch of factor VIII was found and when the patients were traced who received this product it was found that only 50% of them developed antibody.

A recent study has shown that haemophiliacs who received preparations of factor VIII from the United States were six times more likely to have antibodies to HIV than haemophiliacs who had United Kingdom-derived factor VIII. Over 68% of the haemophiliacs who received American factor VIII had HIV antibodies compared to 11% who had United Kingdom-derived factor VIII. This study also established a dose-dependent effect. The greater the number of bottles of contaminated factor VIII the greater the chance of developing antibodies against HIV.

The appearance of AIDS symptoms may be preceded by a relatively long latent period of several years, during which individuals may be infectious. These individuals may therefore provide blood during this period without being aware that they are infected.

An interesting study on the presence of HIV antibody in paid and voluntary blood donors has been reported in Spain. Of 2142 random voluntary blood donors 5 (0.23%) specimens were positive for HIV antibody, whereas 34 (3.3%) of 1020 paid donors were reactive on repeat testing to the presence of HIV antibody. Thus the prevalence of HIV antibody is some 15 times higher in commercial blood than in voluntary blood. Obviously this observation needs confirmation but it may reflect the financial attractions of donating blood to those at risk, particularly intravenous drug abusers.

An article in the *Lancet* in June 1985 expressed the view that blood products prepared from multiple blood donations should be regarded as potentially infectious for AIDS. The authors found that seven out of seventeen reagents prepared from human plasma contained HIV antibodies.

Indications of anti-HIV testing

- Blood transfusions
- Organ transplant donors and semen donors
- Women in high risk groups who are or considering pregnancy
- Patients in renal haemodialysis units
- On request from individuals

A new test to detect the presence of HIV itself rather than antibodies to HIV is under evaluation in blood transfusion centres in the UK. The test, developed by DuPont, uses ELISA to detect specific core protein antigens of HIV called p24. Used in conjunction with current antibody tests the new test will detect the presence of virus in the early stage of infection before antibodies have developed.

HIV INFECTION

In the early stages of infection it is possible, before antibodies are produced, to be antibody-negative but virus-positive. There is thus a wide spectrum of clinical expressions associated with HIV infection ranging from healthy antibody-negative (seronegative) virus-positive persons to antibody-positive (seropositive) patients with fully developed AIDS. Virus-positive, seronegative persons represent the earliest stages of HIV infection with active viral replication and a slowly developing antibody response (see Figure 5.2).

The majority of infected individuals are asymptomatic (healthy carriers). In some patients the acute viral infection is characterized by a glandular fever-like illness with a rash and tender enlarged lymph nodes. The incubation period between infection and development of AIDS is incompletely known and has been found to vary from 6 to 72 months or perhaps longer. During this long latent period the cellular immune system of the patient may be normal although the patient may be infectious to others through sexual intercourse or blood donation. It seems likely that only a few of the infected persons become ill and this is likely to vary with other factors such as immunological stress from recurrent infection, use of recreational drugs, exposure to semen and genetic make-up etc.

The healthy carrier or the person with an acute illness may progress

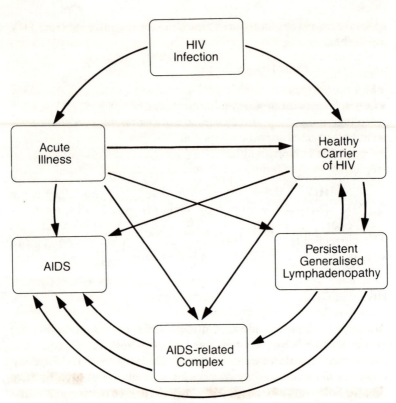

Figure 5.2   HIV-related disease

over a variable time period to one of three conditions (see Figure 5.2)

(a) Persistent Generalized Lymphadenopathy (PGL)

(b) AIDS-related complex (ARC)

(c) Fully blown AIDS

A study in London in 1985 from the Virus Reference Laboratory at the Central Public Health Laboratory examined the occurrence of antibody to HIV in three groups at risk of developing AIDS. Of a large number of homosexuals needing laboratory tests for hepatitis B virus infection in 1984, 34% in London and 5% outside London were positive for HIV antibodies. Obviously these figures cannot be easily extrapolated to the homosexual community as a whole since the group being investigated for hepatitis B infection may be more sexually active than other homosexuals. Furthermore the sample was taken only from those homosexuals who attended sexually transmitted disease clinics. Nevertheless these results provide essential information to help understand the epidemiology of the disease.

In a similar study published at about the same time as that from the Virus Reference Laboratory in London, doctors from the Middlesex Hospital reported the incidence of antibodies to HIV in homosexual/bisexual men in London. The Middlesex group found that the prevalence of antibodies to HIV increased from 3.7% amongst unselected British homosexual men attending the sexually transmitted disease clinic during one week in March 1982, to 31% in those attending during one week in July 1984. About 82% of the seropositive men in 1984 were symptomless or had local symptoms (e.g. urethral discharge). The researchers concluded that HIV was initially imported but is now an endemic sexually transmitted agent and they estimate that as of July 1984 at least 2600 homosexual men in London were probably infected with the AIDS virus. There is therefore a large number of individuals infected with the virus in the United Kingdom, principally in London but also in other metropolitan areas. This will undoubtedly lead to an increase in the number of AIDS patients over the next five years or so.

A similar situation exists in America; the prevalence of HIV antibodies in homosexual men attending a sexually transmitted disease clinic in San Francisco increased from 1% to 65% between 1978 and 1984.

Returning to the Virus Reference Laboratory study the prevalence of antibodies to HIV in haemophiliacs was shown to be higher than that of sexually active homosexuals. About 50% of British haemophiliacs had antibodies against HIV and this is thought to be the result of the use of American factor VIII concentrates. Eventually this risk will be diminished by screening all blood donations for HIV antibodies and heating concentrates to destroy virus. The same study also demonstrated that the prevalence of antibodies in British drug abusers was very small – only about 2.5% had HIV antibodies. This is in marked contrast to the situation in New York where a recent study showed 87% of drug abusers to be infected. These results demonstrate that infection with HIV has rapidly become widespread amongst homosexuals attending sexually transmitted disease clinics and among haemophiliacs receiving pooled blood products. The authors concluded that ... 'every effort must be made by the individuals at immediate risk and those concerned in their medical care to prevent transmission through inoculation of blood, semen and possibly saliva'.

Another interesting study by Dr Richard Tedder at the Middlesex Hospital in London has demonstrated a marked increase in antibodies to HIV in haemophiliacs. Dr Tedder in his research found that antibodies to HIV first occurred in haemophiliacs in 1980. All of these patients had been given commercial factor VIII concentrate imported from the United States. Of samples taken in 1980, 33% were positive for HIV antibodies. This increased to 50% of samples in 1981, 64% in 1982, 66% in 1983 and 64% in 1984. These figures correspond fairly well with the study from the Virus Reference Laboratory discussed above and with recent studies from Denmark and the United States which show prevalence ratios of 64% and 72% respectively for a population with asymptomatic haemophilia. Dr Tedder has commented that widespread infection with HIV is 'laying down an heritage of disease for the future . . . and the problem is not preventing the retrovirus getting into the community, it's already there, but in being able to cope with it'.

At present it is very difficult to provide accurate figures for the total number of persons in this country who are positive for HIV antibodies. If one uses an historical estimate that in the United States 10% of the adult male population are homosexual then from 159 million persons in the United States aged 18 and older there are approximately 8 million homosexuals in America. Given what is already known about the prevalence of HIV antibodies in homosexuals and the potential to spread to other population groups the implications of the presence of AIDS virus in the community are staggering. However these calculations may be erroneous since the natural history of AIDS is still not fully understood. As of January 1987 it is thought that in the UK there are about 30 000–100 000 virus-infected individuals. In the United States about 1.5 million are estimated to be infected with the virus. For every patient with AIDS it is thought that there are 50 other people infected with the AIDS virus.

Another factor to consider is the incidence of HIV antibodies in other risk groups, particularly intravenous drug abusers. A recent Italian study reported in the *Lancet* of 6 July 1985 showed that up to 53% of intravenous drug addicts were seropositive and concluded that 'drug addicts are at a very high risk of HIV infection and that educational and preventative measures should be adopted to prevent further diffusion of HIV infection'.

Finally what are the implications of the widespread introduction of tests for HIV antibody? The test will be principally used to screen blood and blood products and it will be used for diagnostic purposes. Those persons in 'at risk' groups will undoubtedly seek the test. It is possible that an apparently healthy person with a positive HIV test will be denied life insurance and in some cases employment may be terminated. Taken to extreme, governments may require HIV testing before issuing a marriage certificate. We still do not know what it means medically to be HIV positive, only time and further research will tell.

A group of West London genitourinary doctors have stated that the epidemic of HIV infection will produce a significant increase in caseloads presenting to clinic. The author said that their health district alone manages an estimated 5600 male homosexuals annually and the full spectrum of clinical work load remains unknown.

Experts differ in their predictions of how many antibody-positive patients will develop AIDS. The disease has only been recognized since 1981 and it is thought that about 10% of carriers will have AIDS after 5 years, rising to 30% after 7 years. A recent report from Germany has predicted that at least 75% of carriers will develop AIDS. Some AIDS experts in the United States have said privately that all virus-infected individuals will develop AIDS in the long term.

To summarize, a positive antibody result:
- Indicates past infection
- Does not predict whether the individual is still infectious – but it is best to assume so
- Does not predict whether the individual will or will not develop AIDS but as many as 50% may progress to AIDS over 6 to 8 years
- Most persons are infected for life.

RECOMMENDATIONS FOR THE INDIVIDUAL WITH HIV INFECTION

The following guidelines were issued by the WHO in their *Weekly Epidemiological Record* of 25 January 1985.

An individual judged most likely to have an HIV infection should be provided with the following information and advice.

(1) The prognosis for an individual infected with HIV over the long term is not known. However, data available from studies conducted among homosexual men indicate that most persons will remain infected.

(2) Although asymptomatic, these individuals may transmit HIV to others. Regular medical evaluation and follow-up is advised, especially for individuals who develop signs or symptoms suggestive of AIDS.

(3) Refrain from donating blood, plasma, body organs, other tissue, or sperm.

(4) There is a risk of infecting others by sexual intercourse, sharing of needles and, possibly, exposure of others to saliva through oral–genital contact or intimate kissing. The efficacy of condoms in preventing infection with HIV is unproven, but their consistent use may reduce transmission.

(5) Toothbrushes, razors, or other implements that could become contaminated with blood should not be shared.

(6) Women with a seropositive test, or women whose sexual partner is seropositive, are themselves at increased risk of acquiring AIDS. If they become pregnant, their offspring are also at increased risk.

(7) After accidents resulting in bleeding, contaminated surfaces should be cleaned with household bleach freshly diluted 1:10 in water.

(8) Devices that have punctured the skin, such as hypodermic and acupuncture needles, should be steam sterilized by autoclave before re-use or safely discarded. Whenever possible, disposable needles and equipment should be used.

(9) When seeking medical or dental care for intercurrent illness, these persons should inform those responsible for their care of their positive antibody status so that appropriate evaluation can be undertaken and precautions taken to prevent transmission to others.

(10) Testing for HIV antibody should be offered to persons who may have been infected as a result of their contact with seropositive individuals (e.g. sexual partners, persons with whom needles have been shared, infants born to seropositive mothers).

ADVICE FOR GENERAL PRACTITIONERS HANDLING AIDS TESTING

The Chief Medical Officer has provided the following guidelines for managing patients requesting testing for HIV antibodies.

- GPs should give further health education.
- Remind high risk patients not to donate blood or semen or to carry organ donor cards. High risk patients include:
  homosexuals with more than one partner
  injecting drug misusers and their partners
  infected haemophiliacs
  people from areas of high AIDS prevalence.
- Reassure heterosexuals that the chance of past infection is remote unless they have had sexual intercourse without a condom with someone at high risk.
- Male homosexuals with more than one partner and bisexuals need urgent advice on lifestyle. Specialist counselling is available at STD clinics or the Terrence Higgins Trust.
- Drug misusers should be warned about the risks of contracting and transmitting the virus.
- Warn travellers abroad to avoid casual sex with locals. They should try to avoid medical, surgical or dental procedures.
- For others, justification for testing is less clear cut as behaviour modification should be the same whatever the result. A positive antibody test has serious psychological, practical and financial implications.
- After counselling, timing of testing is important. If exposure was recent wait two to three months. If there has been a series of exposures, test on initial presentation and again three months later.

CHAPTER 6

Early symptoms and signs of AIDS

PERSISTENT GENERALIZED LYMPHADENOPATHY (PGL)

Shortly after the first cases of AIDS were described in young male homosexuals it became apparent that another perhaps closely related clinical syndrome was emerging primarily in the same risk groups. Homosexual men at risk for AIDS were developing persistent generalized enlargement of lymph nodes. The syndrome known as persistent generalized lymphadenopathy (PGL) is a precursor or *forme fruste* of AIDS. It is characterized by the prolonged presence of swollen lymph glands in many sites. The glands increase in size, are firm, fully mobile and usually non-tender. They are usually but not always bilateral and remarkably symmetrical – that is the same groups of lymph nodes appear to be affected equally on both sides of the body.

In a normal individual any challenge to the immune system, such as a viral or bacterial infection, can cause swelling of the lymph nodes. In these patients the swelling is a symptom of the underlying problem, not a disease in itself. The lymph nodes are usually tender to touch. After the primary infection has resolved the enlarged glands may decrease to their normal size or they can rarely persist. In a patient with PGL the lymph glands remain enlarged.

Lymph glands can be palpated in a number of places (see Figure 6.1):

(1) Front and back of the neck (cervical)
(2) Behind the ears (occipital)
(3) Over the collar bone (supraclavicular)

(4) Under the arms (axillary)
(5) At the elbows (epitrochlear)
(6) In the groin (inguinal)
(7) Behind the knee (popliteal)

There are literally thousands of lymph glands scattered throughout the body, but they are often too deep to feel by touch. In persistent generalized lymphadenopathy the cervical nodes (both the posterior and anterior), axillary and inguinal lymph nodes are mainly affected. A small proportion of such cases of PGL sometimes progress to the full-blown or fully-expressed AIDS.

The full range of clinical features present in persistent generalized lymphadenopathy includes:

(1) Presence of lymph nodes of 1 cm or greater size for at least 3 months in at least two anatomically distinct sites, other than the inguinal nodes. The mean duration for lymphadenopathy is 18 months and ranges from 3 months to 4 years.

(2) Immunological abnormalities similar to AIDS. Some individuals with PGL have a reversed T-lymphocyte helper to suppressor ratio primarily due to a decrease in T-helper cells.

(3) Absence of acute illness at the onset of lymphadenopathy since some diseases such as glandular fever may also cause swollen glands.

(4) No history of IV drug abuse, recent immunization or other factors which could cause lymphadenopathy.

(5) Lymph node histology on biopsy shows the presence of excess formation of cells – the so-called benign reactive hyperplasia of lymph nodes.

Patients with PGL do not appear seriously ill. They may be asymptomatic or develop one of a range of symptoms such as:

(1) Unexplained fatigue
(2) Fevers
(3) Night sweats
(4) Weight loss
(5) Diarrhoea

The simultaneous appearance of the AIDS epidemic and the PGL

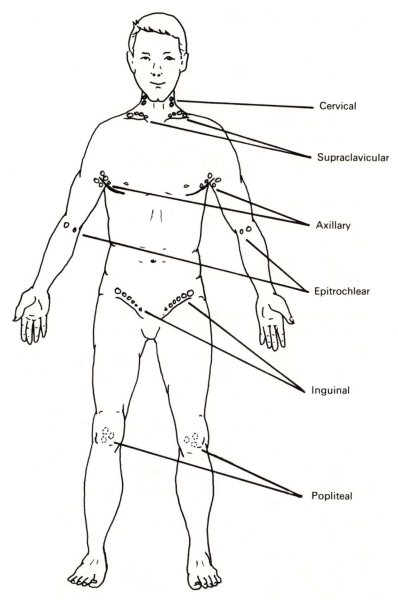

Cervical

Supraclavicular

Axillary

Epitrochlear

Inguinal

Popliteal

Figure 6.1 The lymph glands

syndrome among previously healthy homosexual males suggests a possible association. Similarities between AIDS and the PGL syndrome can be found in:

(1) The epidemiological characteristics of the two syndromes. Both occur primarily in homosexuals with a history of multiple casual or anonymous sexual partners, sexually transmitted diseases and recreational drug use. The average age of onset for both syndromes is in the thirties.

(2) Symptoms described in PGL such as prolonged fatigue, fever, sweats are also seen in AIDS patients.

(3) Cellular immunodeficiencies are similar for both AIDS and PGL but usually much less severe and may be absent altogether in PGL.

(4) About 90% of individuals with PGL are positive for HIV antibodies indicating previous infection with the virus that causes AIDS.

Persistent generalized lymphadenopathy has been described as the AIDS prodrome. However, it is thought that about 30% of patients with PGL go on to develop fully-expressed AIDS, but assessment over longer time periods is needed to provide accurate figures. It also should be remembered that the fully-expressed form of AIDS may occur without a prodromal stage. There are many divergent results from several different studies with regard to the proportion of PGL patients who ultimately develop fully-expressed AIDS. One group of investigators in New York City reported a 17–19% evolution to AIDS while other investigators from San Francisco reported only a 2.5% evolution. It may be that even in these two apparently closely related centres the evolution of the syndrome is one year or more behind in San Francisco compared to New York City. Nevertheless these patients from early studies will provide useful information to help our understanding of the natural host defence mechanisms that are involved in the fight against HIV infection.

Although it is not entirely clear at the present time, the following are positive predictive factors that are required for progression from PGL to AIDS:

(1) Night sweats
(2) Lymphopenia (a decreased lymphocyte count)

(3) The triad of (i) constitutional symptoms (fever, weight loss, fatigue), (ii) splenomegaly (enlarged spleen), and (iii) lymphopenia
(4) Decreased size of lymph nodes with the presence of symptoms
(5) Recurrent herpes zoster (shingles) and oral candidiasis (thrush)

Those seropositive patients that do not develop AIDS may remain carriers of HIV. In addition it should be borne in mind that many cases of unexplained lymphadenopathy in homosexuals are due to the recurrent sexually transmitted diseases which frequently affect this group. For example gonorrhoea, syphilis and cytomegalovirus.

THE AIDS-RELATED COMPLEX (ARC)

The classification of HIV disease is in a state of evolution but the AIDS-related complex (ARC) can be defined as symptomatic infection with HIV with the absence of tumour (e.g. Kaposi's sarcoma) or opportunistic infections. The importance of the separate classification of PGL and ARC reflects the differing prognosis between the relatively benign PGL and the more aggressive ARC. To date, it is thought that about 10% of patients with PGL and about 25% of ARC patients progress to fully-expressed AIDS. But these figures are only provisional and until greater numbers of patients are studied over a longer time period may be grossly underestimated. Furthermore some patients with ARC do not have lymphadenopathy. It is therefore important to try and exclude covert opportunistic infection or tumour in this group of patients.

Symptoms of ARC

- Severe malaise and lethargy
- Weight loss of more than 10% of body weight
- Unexplained diarrhoea for more than one month
- Unexplained fevers and/or night sweats

Clinical signs of ARC

- Oral candidiasis (thrush)
- Oral leucoplakia (white patches on the tongue or cheek)
- Persistent generalized lymphadenopathy (PGL)

- Splenomegaly (enlarged spleen)
- Skin rashes – seborrhoeic eczema and folliculitis

Laboratory abnormalities

(1) Decreased number of T-helper cells.
(2) Decreased ratio of T-helper : T-suppressor lymphocytes.
(3) Anaemia *or* leukopenia *or* thrombocytopenia *or* lymphopenia.
(4) Increased serum globulin levels.
(5) Decreased blastogenic response of lymphocytes to mitogens.
(6) Cutaneous anergy to multiple skin test antigens.
(7) Increased levels of circulating immune complexes.

To be diagnosed as ARC, the patient must have one symptom, one sign and any two or more laboratory abnormalities. The individual must also be free of opportunistic infections and tumour.

Some clinicians do not use the ARC definition or nomenclature. Rather they classify early AIDS patients as PGL with or without symptoms.

EVOLUTION OF PGL AND ARC TO AIDS

There is incomplete data as to what percentage of those HIV antibody-positive individuals will ultimately develop AIDS. It is thought that about 7% per year of infected people go on to develop fully expressed AIDS. Over a 5-year period in different surveys across the world some 10 to 30% of HIV antibody-positive patients have developed AIDS. Over a 10- to 15-year period the percentage may be much higher, perhaps to over 50% or even ultimately to 100%. Only time will tell.

CHAPTER 7

AIDS – The clinical picture

DEFINITION OF AIDS

A precise definition of the Acquired Immune Deficiency Syndrome is still not available because relatively little is known about the basic disease process and the resulting immunological defects. The working definition from the Communicable Disease Surveillance Centre at Collindale adopted from the Centers for Disease Control (CDC) in Atlanta in the United States is as follows:

For the limited purposes of epidemiological surveillance a case of acquired immune deficiency syndrome is defined as one in which a person has

(1) A reliably diagnosed disease that is at least moderately indicative of an underlying cellular immune deficiency (such as an opportunistic infection, or Kaposi's sarcoma in a person aged less than 60 years)

(2) No known underlying cause of cellular immune deficiency nor any other cause of reduced resistance reported to be associated with that disease.

The definition has also been accepted by many countries and by the World Health Organization (WHO) collaborating centre for AIDS. The full definition and modified case definition of AIDS from the CDC is provided in Appendix 5. This shows the guidelines for natural reporting of AIDS in the United States through the CDC. In particular it brings into the definition of AIDS the HIV antibody status of an individual.

Opportunistic infections that are indicative of AIDS must be:

(1) Suggestive of a cellular immune deficiency
(2) Sufficiently uncommon in an immunologically normal popu-
    lation to be useful as a discriminating test.

Strict application of the criteria in the Centers for Disease Control
definition has ensured reliable and reproducible information about
the AIDS epidemic. At the same time, however, it has only identified
the most severe and later manifestations of the disease and has
probably resulted in an underestimation of the size and severity of
the HIV problem.

SPECTRUM OF DISORDERS SEEN IN AIDS

It is hoped that in the near future a more accurate definition of AIDS
will be available based on serological criteria, e.g. presence of HIV
antibodies and/or markers of the immunological abnormalities
characteristic of AIDS. In addition, now that the AIDS virus has
been identified it should also be possible to define individuals who
are asymptomatic or symptomatic carriers of the disease and those
individuals who later develop the fully-expressed syndrome.

The presence of antibody to the HIV virus in 'at risk' patients has
shown an alarming increase over the last 2–3 years. In London in
1982 only about 2% of the homosexual population had antibodies
to HIV. In 1985 however this figure is nearer to 30%. Thus extra-
polating this figure it would appear that about 30% of homosexuals
in London have been infected with HIV. In San Francisco in 1980
only about 10% of homosexuals had antibodies to HIV but in 1984,
70% of homosexuals had antibodies to the AIDS virus.

There is now an increasing recognition of a far higher incidence
of less severe illnesses in individuals known to be at an increased risk
for AIDS (Figure 7.1).

Additional conditions which occur with increased frequency in
AIDS patients include:

(1) A range of malignant neoplasms:
    (a) Lymphomas (tumours arising from lymphatic tissue)
        ● Burkitt's lymphoma (which is associated with the Epstein–
          Barr virus)

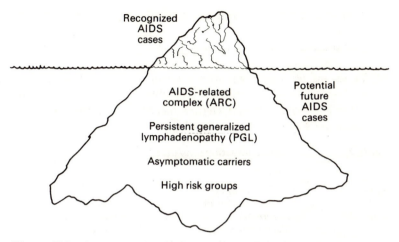

Figure 7.1   Spectrum of disorders seen in AIDS – the iceberg effect

- Undifferentiated non-Hodgkin's lymphoma
- Cerebral lymphoma
    (b) Squamous cell carcinoma of the oral cavity and anus.

(2) Autoimmune conditions:
    (a) Idiopathic thrombocytopenic purpura (ITP). (A rare disease which is characterized by bleeding from blood capillaries in the skin, nose, uterus and alimentary tract.)
    (b) Autoimmune haemolytic anaemia. (An abnormally rapid breakdown of red blood cells which causes anaemia and sometimes jaundice.)

(3) Condyloma acuminata (genital warts) of the genital and peri-anal area. These are seen more frequently in AIDS patients and are often unresponsive to conventional therapy. However genital warts are not often a serious problem.

CLINICAL FEATURES OF AIDS

The signs and symptoms which may suggest AIDS are:

(1) Profound fatigue persisting for several weeks with no obvious cause.

(2) Swollen lymph glands usually bilaterally in the cervical, axillary and inguinal regions.

(3) Unexpected weight loss of more than 10 pounds (4.5 kg) in two months.

(4) Persistent fever or night sweats lasting for several weeks. The pathogens most frequently responsible for causing a fever are cytomegalovirus, *Mycobacterium tuberculosis* or atypical mycobacteria (See Table 7.1 for details).

Table 7.1   Opportunistic infections in AIDS

	Common	Uncommon
Viral	Herpes simplex	Herpes zoster
	Cytomegalovirus	Polyoma virus
Bacterial	*Salmonella typhimurium*	*M. avium intracellulare*
	M. tuberculosis	*Legionella*
	M. xenopi/kanasii/avium intracellulare	
Fungal	*Candida albicans*	*Histoplasma capsulatum*
	Cryptococcus neoformans	
	Tinea species	
Protozoal	*Pneumocystis carinii*	*Isopora* species
	Toxoplasma gondii	
	Cryptosporidium species	

(5) Persistent shortness of breath and non-productive cough of several weeks duration.

(6) Skin disease – Kaposi's sarcoma – new pink to purple blotches, flat or raised, like a bruise or a blood blister. These can be anywhere on the skin including the mouth or eyelids.

A number of other skin complaints are common among AIDS patients including fungal infections, folliculitis and eczema. The reason for eczematous and infected lesions of the skin is unclear but it may reflect changes in the organisms on the skin surface or the host's reaction to them.

Shingles (herpes zoster) is also very common, occurring in about 25% of patients.

(7) Alimentary tract

(a) Thrush – AIDS may present with oral and oesophageal candidiasis. Oral thrush is very common in AIDS and in other patients indicates an increased likelihood of developing AIDS.

(b) Diarrhoea – usually profuse and chronic and may be caused by cryptosporidiosis, cytomegalovirus or atypical mycobacteria (see Tables 7.1 and 7.2 for details)
(8) Central nervous system – lethargy, depression and sometimes in late stages dementia. It is thought that HIV may directly infect

Table 7.2 Opportunistic infections common in AIDS

Agents	Sites of infection	Most common clinical manifestations in AIDS
Protozoan agents		
Pneumocystis carinii	Lungs	Pneumonia
Toxoplasma gondii	Brain	Abscess
	Lymph nodes, blood	Disseminated infections*
Giardia lamblia	Intestine and biliary tract	Diarrhoea
Entamoeba histolytica	Intestine, liver	Diarrhoea
Cryptosporidium enteritis	Intestine	Diarrhoea
Viruses		
Herpes simplex	Mouth, genitals, buttocks, hands	Ulcerative lesions
	Brain	Disseminated infections*
Cytomegalovirus	Lungs	Pneumonia
	Lymph nodes, liver, blood	Disseminated infections*
	Eye	Retinitis
	Intestine	Colitis
Epstein–Barr	Blood, brain, liver, lymph nodes	Disseminated infections*
Bacterial agents		
Salmonella	Intestine	Diarrhoea
(various)	Blood	Septicaemia
Shigella flexneri	Intestine	Diarrhoea
Mycobacterium tuberculosis	Lung	Tuberculosis
Mycobacterium avium-intracellulare	Liver, lymph nodes, spleen, bone marrow	Lymphadenopathy and disseminated infections*

[*table continued overleaf*]

* Disseminated infections describes the involvement of lungs, multiple lymph nodes or other internal organs.

Table 7.2—contd.

Agents	Sites of infection	Most common clinical manifestations in AIDS
Fungal agents		
Cryptococcus neoformans	Brain Lungs	Meningitis Pneumonia
Cryptococcus neoformans	Skin	Disseminated infections*
Aspergillosis	Lung, brain	Pneumonia and disseminated infections*
Histoplasmosis	Lung, skin, lymph nodes	Pneumonia and disseminated infections*
Candida albicans	Mouth, throat, oesophagus	Oral thrush and oesophagitis

* Disseminated infections describes the involvement of lungs, multiple lymph nodes or other internal organs.

nervous tissue (neurotropic) and cause an acute or subacute encephalitis (AIDS-encephalopathy) which may account for central nervous system disorders in AIDS.

As early as 1982 it was noticed that patients with fully developed AIDS were developing a dementing illness. This was characterized by a change in personality, loss of short and long term memory and an inability to concentrate. Computerized (CT) X-ray scanning of the brain reveals a marked atrophy of both white and grey matter. Recently, it has been demonstrated that the genetic material from HIV has been found in brain cells. This condition, termed the AIDS encephalopathy, therefore represents a primary AIDS virus infection of the central nervous system and affects about 40% of patients with AIDS. The initial presentation may be extremely subtle – usually short term memory loss but even when quite advanced it may be difficult to document.

At present there is no effective treatment for the AIDS encephalopathy and it is not certain whether all those individuals infected with HIV will develop this condition over several years.

Neurological effects of HIV infection:

- Encephalopathy
- Personality changes
- Lack of concentration

- Disorientation
- Impairment of speech
- Impairment of vision

Also the opportunistic pathogens toxoplasmosis (a protozoa), cryptococcus (a fungus) and cytomegalovirus invade the central nervous system and may produce focal, diffuse and retinal lesions respectively (see Table 7.2 for details).

The devastating nature of the immune deficiency in AIDS renders previously healthy individuals susceptible to a broad range of opportunistic infections and malignancies. These are the outward and major manifestations which define the disease.

The spectrum of opportunistic infections includes protozoans, viruses, bacteria and fungal agents. Table 7.2 shows the range of

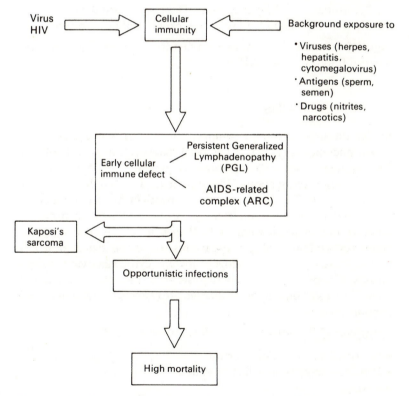

Figure 7.2 An hypothesis for the development of AIDS

opportunistic infective agents that have been isolated from AIDS patients, and the wide range of diseases these agents may cause in a patient with AIDS.

Kaposi's sarcoma is the most frequently diagnosed malignancy in AIDS. The prognosis for AIDS patients with this tumour and no evidence of opportunistic infections is much more favourable than those with *Pneumocystis carinii* pneumonia. The cause of death in AIDS patients is nearly always due to overwhelming infection rather than uncontrolled malignancy.

Thus an AIDS patient may present to hospital as an acute admission to the following specialists:

(1) Chest physicians – Pneumonia and severe chest infections
(2) Gastroenterologists – Severe diarrhoea
(3) Dermatologists – Kaposi's sarcoma
(4) Neurologists and psychiatrists – Depression and dementia
(5) General physicians – Fever or pyrexia of unknown origin

Figure 7.2 summarizes the various factors involved in the development of fully-expressed AIDS.

Chest disease in AIDS

By far the most common complication of AIDS is *Pneumocystis carinii* pneumonia (PCP). It has been diagnosed in almost 94% of haemophiliac cases, 73% of drug-user patients and 55% of homosexual cases. Overall about 58% of patients with AIDS develop this infection and PCP is the major cause of death in AIDS patients. PCP has caused about three-quarters of British and American deaths. Another interesting feature of PCP seen in a setting of immunodeficiency is that multiple organisms are often detected in the lungs. These coexisting pathogens include cytomegalovirus, herpes viruses, toxoplasma, and tuberculosis and *Legionella* bacteria (see below). In addition Kaposi's sarcoma also affects the lung in a small proportion of patients with AIDS.

Symptoms of Pneumocystis carinii *pneumonia* (*PCP*)

● Shortness of breath on exertion
● Persistent dry non-productive cough
● Fever
● Mild pleuritic chest pain

Signs
- There may be none
- Increased rate of respiration
- Crackles at lung base
- Central cyanosis (bluish discolouration of the skin, lips and nail beds caused by insufficient oxygen in the blood)

Organisms
- *Pneumocystis carinii*
- Cytomegalovirus
- Mycobacteria
- *Candida albicans*
- Herpes
- *Legionella*

Investigations
- Chest X-ray – characteristic findings – interstitial lung shadowing
- Fibre-optic bronchoscopy with transbronchial biopsy of alveolar tissue
- Blood gas analysis and other lung function tests

CAUSES OF DEATH IN AIDS

	Percentage
Respiratory	60%
pneumocystis	
cytomegalovirus	
bacterial	
Central nervous system	20%
toxoplasma	
encephalopathy	
Kaposi's sarcoma	10%
Other	10%

NEW CLASSIFICATION FOR HIV INFECTION

On 23 May 1986 the Centers for Disease Control proposed a classification system for HIV infection primarily applicable to public health purposes, including disease reporting and surveillance, epidemiologic studies, prevention and control activities, and public health policy and planning.

The system classifies the manifestations of HIV infection into four

Table 7.3   Summary of classification system for HIV-associated disease

Group I.	Acute infection
Group II.	Asymptomatic infection*
Group III.	Persistent generalized lymphadenopathy*
Group IV.	Other disease
Subgroup A.	Constitutional disease
Subgroup B.	Neurologic disease
Subgroup C.	Secondary infectious diseases
Category C-1.	Specified secondary infectious diseases listed in the CDC surveillance definition for AIDS†
Category C-2.	Other specified secondary infectious diseases
Subgroup D.	Secondary cancers†
Subgroup E.	Other conditions

* Patients in Groups II and III may be subclassified on the basis of a laboratory evaluation
† Includes those patients whose clinical presentation fulfils the definition of AIDS used by CDC for national reporting. (See Appendix 5.)

mutually exclusive groups, designated by Roman numerals I–IV (Table 7.3). The classification system applies only to patients diagnosed as having HIV infection.

Group I includes patients with transient signs and symptoms that appear at the time of, or shortly after, initial infection with HIV as identified by laboratory studies. Defined as glandular fever-like illness.

Group II includes patients who have no signs or symptoms of HIV infection. Patients in this category may be subclassified based on whether haematological and/or immunological laboratory studies have been done and whether results are abnormal in a manner consistent with the effects of HIV infection.

Group III includes patients with persistent generalized lymphadenopathy, but without findings that would lead to classification in Group IV. Patients in this category may be subclassified based on the results of laboratory studies as in Group I.

Group IV includes patients with clinical symptoms and signs of HIV infection other than or in addition to lymphadenopathy. Patients in this group are assigned to *one or more* subgroups based on clinical findings (Table 7.3). In Subgroup C the patients are divided further into two categories: *Category C-1* includes patients with symptomatic or invasive disease due to one of 12 specified secondary infectious diseases listed in the surveillance definition of AIDS (see Appendix 5). *Category C-2* includes patients with systemic or invasive disease due to one of six other specified secondary infectious diseases (see Appendix 5).

CHAPTER 8

Kaposi's sarcoma

Kaposi's sarcoma as a manifestation of AIDS occurs in about 25% of all AIDS cases; about 10% of this proportion develop this tumour with an opportunistic infection. The different risk groups for AIDS, however, appear to have different susceptibilities for developing this cancer. In homosexual patients the risk is about 5 times that of a patient from any of the other risk groups. About 40% of homosexual AIDS patients develop Kaposi's sarcoma. The reason for such a prevalence in homosexuals is unclear, but it is believed that the sarcoma is caused by an as yet unidentified opportunistic virus widespread in the homosexual community but rare in other groups.

DEFINITION

Kaposi's sarcoma is a cancer of the skin and connective tissues. The exact cell of origin is not known although it is believed to arise from endothelial cells such as the cells which line blood vessels. Malignant transformation causes the inner wall of small blood vessels to become stippled with spindle-shaped tumour cells. A similar picture may be seen when Kaposi's sarcoma involves lymph nodes and internal organs. The continued growth of the tumour may produce lymphatic obstruction and as a result the affected limbs become swollen and internal organs may become congested and enlarged. The tumour does not metastasize, it is multifocal and involves numerous sites with a predilection for the gastrointestinal tract, from the mouth to the anus. Therefore in many cases the tumour remains localized and is of no problem to the patient.

Kaposi's sarcoma is not a new disease although in the United States it was certainly very rare before 1978 with only 0.02–0.06 cases per 100 000 population, well below 1% of all cancers. However, in certain settings Kaposi's sarcoma was known to be far more frequent and is characterized by two types: classical Kaposi's sarcoma and African Kaposi's sarcoma.

(1) Classical Kaposi's sarcoma

This occurs in elderly men, over 50 years, of Ashkenazi, Jewish or Mediterranean descent. Kaposi's sarcoma was initially identified in this group in 1872, by an Austrian dermatologist Dr Moritz Kohn Kaposi who described it as an 'idiopathic multiple pigmented sarcoma of the skin'. For over 50 years after Kaposi's original description researchers were mainly concerned with the epidemiological, clinical and pathological aspects of the disease. The last five years have seen a remarkable increase in prevalence of this disease particularly associated with homosexual men.

Clinical features
The disease course is generally indolent and it rarely affects the internal organs. Purple or blue patches appear mostly on the skin of the lower extremities, especially the feet although lesions can appear anywhere on the skin or mucous membranes and in the gastrointestinal tract. There may be just one or hundreds of lesions and they are often associated with surrounding oedema, signifying tumour infiltration into lymphatics or veins. These skin lesions often coalesce forming large plaques or nodules and may ulcerate. Patients often die of illnesses unrelated to the neoplasm. There may be an increased incidence of secondary malignancies, particularly lymphoma among patients with classical Kaposi's sarcoma.

Average survival time in this group of elderly patients is 8–13 years which is comparable to age-matched controls without Kaposi's sarcoma.

Table 8.1   Comparison of clinical features of Kaposi's sarcoma

	Classical (sporadic)	African (endemic)	AIDS (epidemic)
Skin lesion	Legs, feet	Extremities	Widely dispersed
Mucosal involvement	Rare	Rare	Common (oral, anal)
Lymph node involvement	Rare	Uncommon	Frequent
Response to treatment	Excellent	Excellent	Poor
Indolent course	Common	Common	Unusual

(2) African Kaposi's sarcoma

In Africa, particularly Zaire, Kenya and Tanzania which are predominantly hill and open bush country, Kaposi's sarcoma is endemic. This cancer is 200 times more frequent than in the United States and accounts for about 10% of all neoplasms. The highest incidence is in Zaire. The cancer commonly affects African children in the first decade of life with an equal incidence among males and females. It also occurs with increasing frequency in men over 25 years of age.

Clinical features
Endemic Kaposi's sarcoma tends to be more aggressive and fatal than the classical type of Kaposi's sarcoma found in elderly men of Jewish or Mediterranean origin. Spread to the internal organs is common and death inevitably occurs within three years of diagnosis. Several studies have shown that the majority of patients with AIDS-related disorders in Uganda and Zambia have HIV antibodies.

A comparison of some of the clinical features of the various types of Kaposi's sarcoma is shown in Table 8.1.

KAPOSI'S SARCOMA AND AIDS

The development of Kaposi's sarcoma in AIDS patients is not the first time that this cancer has occurred in a setting of immune deficiency. It has been known for many years that individuals with kidney transplants, congenital immunodeficiencies or systemic diseases treated with immunosuppressive drugs have a greatly increased risk for developing Kaposi's sarcoma. This has suggested that immunosuppression has a permissive effect on the development of Kaposi's sarcoma.

(1) Aetiology of Kaposi's sarcoma

The cause of Kaposi's sarcoma is still unknown. The great regional variation in prevalence and the clustering of cases in Africa support an infectious aetiology. An association with cytomegalovirus has in particular been investigated. Cytomegalovirus DNA has been found in African Kaposi's sarcoma tissue and in cell lines derived from tumour tissue.

Cytomegalovirus is an extremely common virus. More than 90% of active homosexuals have evidence of exposure, and transplant recipients receiving immunosuppressive drugs are at increased risk of CMV infection as well as Kaposi's sarcoma. However, it has also been noted that while African Kaposi's sarcoma patients have high antibody blood levels to CMV these are not significantly different from controls from the same region. There is as yet no direct proven connection between CMV and the genesis of Kaposi's sarcoma.

The integrity of the immune system may be important in the development of Kaposi's sarcoma. Possibly immune suppression such as that caused by HIV is required before the specific factor causing Kaposi's sarcoma can induce its effect. Several cases of spontaneous regression have been reported in transplantation patients following discontinuation of the immunosuppressive therapy and recently there has been reported one case of spontaneous regression of AIDS-related Kaposi's sarcoma.

Genetic host factors may also be involved. There is some evidence that both AIDS-associated Kaposi's sarcoma and the classic type are related to a particular tissue type. However, studies in AIDS patients who have developed only opportunistic infections have not as yet demonstrated any specific genetic links.

(2) Clinical features

The most common presentation of Kaposi's sarcoma in AIDS patients is isolated skin lesions with early involvement of lymph nodes and viscera. Skin lesions range from tiny faint pink, slightly raised lesions to deep purple or blue nodules 1 cm or more in size; they rarely are bigger than 5 cm in diameter. These lesions are generally painless, at first often resembling a small bruise, and may occur anywhere on the body, affecting the limbs, trunk and head and neck area.

It is thought that as many as 50% of patients have small or large intestine involvement which in itself is indicative of a greater tumour load in the body. Lesions in the oropharynx are relatively frequent as well. These are usually asymptomatic and cause only minor problems.

For some AIDS patients Kaposi's sarcoma is a rapidly progressive disease with involvement of virtually every organ. Lesions of the head and neck may be particularly disfiguring. Despite the aggressive nature of this cancer it is rarely fatal, most AIDS patients succumb first to severe opportunistic infection.

(3) Staging of Kaposi's sarcoma

Kaposi's sarcoma has been classified into four clinical stages (see Table 8.2):

Stage I corresponds to the common type of Kaposi's sarcoma seen in elderly patients, usually males. Stage II identifies the florid, locally aggressive lesions of patients with the African type of Kaposi's

Table 8.2 Staging of Kaposi's sarcoma

Stage I	– Limited cutaneous – Patients with less than 10 skin lesions or lesions restricted to a single anatomical site, e.g. one extremity. Locally indolent
Stage II	– Cutaneous locally aggressive – lesions in more than one anatomical region e.g. head, trunk and extremities
Stage III	– Generalized mucocutaneous ± lymph nodes
Stage IV	– Generalized skin lesions and visceral involvement

sarcoma often involving regional lymph nodes. Stages III and IV identify the generalized disseminated form of Kaposi's sarcoma seen commonly in North American male homosexuals. Since about half of all patients with Kaposi's sarcoma associated with AIDS have visceral involvement, the majority of patients have stage III or IV disease.

The clinical staging allows the physician to define the severity of the disease and the eventual outcome. Since stages III and IV represent more advanced disease they have a poor prognosis compared with stages I and II of Kaposi's sarcoma.

Patients are also staged according to the presence or absence of symptoms.

Subclass A – Asymptomatic
Subclass B – Fevers, weight loss of 15 lb or 10% bodyweight, diarrhoea without known cause

The presence of criteria given in subclass B further reduces the prognosis and response rate. The staging system may therefore enable physicians to identify patients requiring early aggressive chemotherapy or more conventional radiotherapy.

(4) Tests used for staging and diagnosis of Kaposi's sarcoma

(a) Skin: photographs and biopsy of lesion/s
(b) Lymph nodes: biopsy of accessible nodes and special X-rays (computerized tomography – CT scanning) of the abdomen and pelvis
(c) Gastrointestinal tract: fibreoptic endoscopy and colonoscopy with appropriate biopsy are more sensitive than barium contrast studies in localizing tumour
(d) Lung: fibreoptic bronchoscopy when chest X-ray is abnormal
(e) Liver: radioisotope or CT scan
(f) Bone: bone scan if serum alkaline phosphatase is raised
(g) Bone marrow: biopsy if blood count is abnormal
(h) Brain: computerized axial tomography (CAT scan)

A comparison of the epidemiology of African Kaposi's sarcoma and the neoplasm in AIDS patients does, however, show close similarities (see Table 8.3). Both are highly area-specific, are far more

Table 8.3 Comparison of the epidemiology of African Kaposi's sarcoma and AIDS Kaposi's sarcoma

	African Kaposi's sarcoma	AIDS Kaposi's sarcoma
Sex ratio (M:F)	13:1	14:1
Age	Small peak 2–3 y Increase after 20 y Median 25–40 y	Small peak 1–2 y Increase after 20 y Median 30–39 y
Geographical distribution	Equatorial Africa Highly area specific	USA, Europe, Africa Highly area specific
Social distribution	All tribal groups Upper/lower classes	All ethnic groups All classes
Infectivity	Clustering	Clustering Sexually transmitted Blood-borne
Associated infections	Cytomegalovirus Herpes simplex virus Epstein–Barr virus Hepatitis B virus *E. histolytica*	Cytomegalovirus Herpes simplex virus Epstein–Barr virus Hepatitis B virus *E. histolytica* Syphilis
Opportunist infections	Not recorded/? missed	50% *Pneumocystis carinii* pneumonia 25% other

common in men particularly over 20 years old, and show evidence of past exposure to an identical range of viral and protozoal infections. Unfortunately, there is no accurate information available on the incidence of opportunistic infections in Africa whereas over 50% of AIDS patients develop these infections. This lack of evidence may be attributable to two factors:

(a) In Africa the prevalence of infectious diseases is high and sudden death through such diseases in a young age group is not uncommon.

(b) The standard of health care is such that an opportunist infection in a young patient may easily pass unrecognized.

The epidemiological similarities are further strengthened by the immunological changes common to both. A recent Zambian study showed that patients with endemic Kaposi's sarcoma had decreased ratios of T-lymphocyte helper cells to T-suppressor cells as do patients with AIDS.

In view of these close similarities in epidemiology it has been speculated that African Kaposi's sarcoma may also be involved in the outbreak of AIDS. AIDS cases have been reported in Europeans who have had sexual contact with Africans and individuals living in Central Africa. Two cases of an AIDS-like syndrome which were diagnosed retrospectively in two female patients from Zaire have received particular interest because they precede the first documented American cases by several years. AIDS may, therefore, have been present in Africa before it was present in the United States.

It has been proposed that the endemic Kaposi's sarcoma seen in Africa is actually part of the Acquired Immune Deficiency Syndrome with opportunistic infections being missed more frequently in this setting. On the basis of epidemiological similarities it is suggested that transmission of AIDS in Africa may also be by homosexual contact. Recent evidence however suggests that AIDS in Africa is transmitted by heterosexual contact (see Chapter 2). The current AIDS epidemic may have resulted from the spread of this disease outside its contained rural African setting to other parts of Africa and in particular to the United States and Europe.

Prognosis for patients with Kaposi's sarcoma

The life-expectancy of AIDS patients with opportunistic infections is about eight months; none so far have survived for as long as three years. For AIDS patients with Kaposi's sarcoma the average life-expectancy is about 16 months and only about 25% have survived for two years. Mortality rates are highest for those patients with both opportunistic infections and Kaposi's sarcoma.

There are, however, many variables to consider to establish prognosis and predict survival in patients with Kaposi's sarcoma. These include:

(a) Clinical features, for example staging and clinical status
(b) Viral antibody status
(c) Immunological parameters.

About 80% of those patients with Kaposi's sarcoma who do not have an opportunistic infection will be alive at 28 months.

CHAPTER 9

Treatment and management of AIDS

The main goal in the treatment of AIDS is to simultaneously suppress the virus and build up the immune system in the patient.

Patients with AIDS usually require intensive medical investigation and nursing care. They may be in and out of hospital at regular intervals over a period of 2–3 years. Thus the management of AIDS patients is very expensive. In the United States the cost of treating an AIDS patient is estimated at around $150 000. In the United Kingdom the cost is probably around £10 000 but there are no accurate figures. Certainly when all patients with minor illnesses caused by HIV infection are considered along with the counselling and contact tracing required this exercise becomes very expensive. It has been estimated that in Britain the cost of treating victims of AIDS and of controlling the spread of the disease is about £20 million a year.

To date, there is no vaccine or any other drug available which can prevent someone developing AIDS. It is very difficult to make a vaccine against a specific virus – a good example of this is the vaccines available for influenza. These are usually very virus-specific and a small change in the nature of the virus renders the vaccine ineffective. It is thought that a similar situation exists with the AIDS virus and it may prove difficult to produce a highly effective vaccine. Various experts have predicted that a commercial vaccine will not be available before 1990. Since the genetic make-up of HIV is known it may make the production of a vaccine easier but so far only one retrovirus vaccine has been produced – the feline leukaemia virus vaccine. The

AIDS virus has proved difficult to make a vaccine against for several reasons:

(a) HIV is able to mutate rapidly, changing the structure of its identifying surface antigens so frequently that the immune system is unable to produce antibodies fast enough to keep up with the virus. Thus a vaccine could produce a similar situation to the body's own response to the AIDS virus – antibodies are produced but are unable to neutralize the invading viruses. An AIDS researcher has stated 'The chance of going to a lab and creating something nature hasn't done yet is slim'.

(b) HIV is able to fuse helper T-cells and move from one to another without returning to the bloodstream. Within cells the virus is safe from neutralizing antibodies whether produced naturally or stimulated by a vaccine.

(c) HIV is in itself destructive to the immune system by destroying helper T-cells and this impairs the production of neutralizing antibodies.

(d) There are also some important safety considerations – the vaccine should produce no risk of AIDS or immune dysfunction.

(e) Clinical trials of the vaccine will take time since the long incubation period of HIV might imply years of clinical trial to establish safety and efficacy.

(f) There are also potential problems of product liability – if pharmaceutical or related companies have to bear liability they would probably not produce a vaccine.

The management of AIDS patients can be conveniently divided into:

(1) Treatment of opportunistic infections
(2) Treatment of Kaposi's sarcoma
(3) Treatment of the underlying immune deficiency syndrome
(4) Anti-HIV agents
(5) Other treatment – plasmapheresis, bone marrow transplantation and leukocyte transfusion
(6) General management and precautions when dealing with AIDS patients
(7) Counselling of AIDS patients – When a Friend has AIDS, Taking Care of Yourself and Others
(8) Safe sex guidelines

(1) TREATMENT OF OPPORTUNISTIC INFECTIONS

(a) Candida infection (candidiasis) is a ubiquitous infection of people with AIDS affecting the mouth, oesophagus and occasionally the skin around the armpits, groin and rectum. *Candida albicans* is a fungus (usually called thrush) that is one of the normal inhabitants of the skin, mouth and vagina of healthy individuals. Symptoms and signs of oral candida infection are white or cream coloured patches or plaques on the tongue, lips, throat and inside of the mouth. It may cause swelling, redness, changes in taste and a painful or burning sensation. Diagnosis can be confirmed by taking a scraping and examination under the microscope. Symptoms of oesophageal candidiasis include sore throat, difficulty in swallowing and pain behind the sternum (breastbone). A series of X-rays including a barium swallow or endoscopy confirm the diagnosis.

Treatment of oral thrush is usually with oral liquids or suspensions of antifungal drugs: Nystatin 100 000 units per ml rinsed around the mouth, gargled and swallowed four times a day keeps thrush under control. If there is no effect with oral liquids, tablets of ketoconazole may be used particularly for oesophageal candidiasis. If the infection does not respond or is more widespread, treatment with an intravenous antifungal agent, amphotericin B, may be required.

(b) Herpes. There are three types of herpes virus:

   (i) Herpes simplex type 1 (HSV1) – causes cold sores on the mouth and face.

  (ii) Herpes simplex type 2 (HSV2) – causes painful sores and ulcers around the genitals and anus. HSV2 is sexually transmitted and after oral candidiasis is the commonest infection seen in people with AIDS.

 (iii) Herpes zoster – the same virus causes chickenpox in children and remains dormant in the body and may reappear in adults as herpes zoster or shingles. It is characterized by painful blisters and ulcers on the skin that follow nerve pathways. Although commonly seen in AIDS-related complex (ARC) herpes zoster is uncommon in fully developed AIDS.

All herpes viruses may lie dormant for months or years in nerves and then flare up as a result of stress, trauma, infection or immunosuppression. Herpes infections may disseminate and affect larger areas of skin and major organs such as the lungs, brain and gastrointestinal tract.

Treatment is with an anti-herpes preparation called acyclovir. Mild cases may be controlled by oral administration; disseminated infections require intravenous acyclovir. Fortunately, acyclovir has very few side effects and is generally well tolerated.

(c) *Pneumocystis carinii* pneumonia (PCP). PCP is the most common cause of death in patients with AIDS. There is however specific chemotherapy which initially is highly effective in this type of pneumonia. AIDS patients with PCP require longer courses and higher doses of medication than those patients with PCP as a result of cancer chemotherapy or organ transplantation. The drugs are used either alone or in combination according to the following regime:

- Co-trimoxazole ('Septrin', 'Bactrim'). Sixteen tablets per day for individual doses 21 days or a similar dose given intravenously

- Pentamidine isethionate 4 mg/kg/day. Can only be administered either by the intramuscular or intravenous route

These drugs are not without problems since adverse reactions are common. Up to 80% of patients given this high dose regimen of co-trimoxazole develop a rash which in some cases is severe and necessitates change of therapy. About 50% of patients given pentamidine develop a transient deterioration in kidney function. Painful sterile abscesses at the injection sites may also occur and patients may refuse further injections.

Other broad spectrum antibiotics including penicillin, erythromycin and the tetracyclines have no activity against PCP.

Pentamidine is available free of charge from the Centers for Disease Control in Atlanta and its increased use in the last two years has reflected the incidence of AIDS in the United States.

The mortality from a first attack of PCP is about 30% – that is, 70% of patients with PCP respond to initial therapy with either co-trimoxazole or pentamidine. However survival from subsequent episodes of infection is much worse and the mean survival time for a patient with PCP is about thirty weeks. The two-year survival time after one episode of PCP is zero.

Interestingly if the patient with PCP also has Kaposi's sarcoma his overall survival time appears to be prolonged to about sixty weeks. For Kaposi's sarcoma alone the overall survival time is about 125 weeks. The quality of life, however, of a patient with PCP is variable – in one study about 40% of patients spent more than half the time from diagnosis to death in hospital.

(d) *Toxoplasmosis gondii*-like pneumocystis is an opportunistic protozoan that becomes evident as an individual's immunity becomes compromised. The commonest clinical problems of toxoplasmosis in AIDS is infection of the central nervous system causing encephalitis and brain abscesses and results in rapid deterioration. Treatment is with sulphadiazine and pyrimethamine (Fansidar). Treatment is needed for many months and repeated regularly perhaps for the lifetime of the patient. The chance of a relapse is high.

(e) Cryptococcal infection. The fungus *Cryptococcus neoformans* mainly causes meningitis in immunocompromised individuals. It may also affect other organs such as the lungs, bone and genito-urinary system. Patients with cryptococcal meningitis may present with a persistent headache, mild fever and sometimes blurred vision. There may be subtle changes in cerebral function including confusion and decreased concentration.

Cryptococcal meningitis is diagnosed by finding the fungus in cerebrospinal fluid, sputum, urine and blood.

Treatment is with antifungal drugs such as 5-flucytosine and amphotericin B. Relapse is common once treatment is finished but may occur several months later.

(f) Amoebiasis and giardiasis. *Entamoeba histolytica* (a protozoan which causes amoebiasis) and *Giardia lamblia* (a protozoan which causes giardiasis) cause what is described as the 'Gay Bowel Syndrome'. Clinically, these protozoal infections present with diarrhoea, bloating and excess intestinal gas (flatus) and are common complaints seen in the homosexual community in America but occur less commonly in the United Kingdom. Although these organisms are common in homosexual men they usually pose no problems to the patient with AIDS. Treatment is with appropriate antiprotozoal drugs or metronidazole.

(g) Cryptosporidiosis. Cryptosporidiosis, a protozoan parasite, has

Table 9.1 Treatment of opportunistic infections in patients with AIDS

Effective therapy is available for:
  Pneumocystis carinii
  Toxoplasma gondii
  Candida species
  Cryptococcus neoformans   Relapses are common
  Mycobacterium tuberculosis
  Herpex simplex
  Herpes zoster

Effective therapy is not currently available for:
  Cryptosporidium
  Mycobacterium avium-intracellulare
  Cytomegalovirus
  Epstein–Barr virus

only recently (since 1976) been recognized as a problem in humans. Previously it was a cause of diarrhoea in turkeys, snakes, calves and lambs and some rodents. It was occasionally seen in slaughterhouse workers or vets who develop a self-limiting diarrhoea that requires no therapy. In AIDS patients the diarrhoea is often chronic, watery and very profuse or voluminous amounting to 10–12 litres per day. Bowel movement frequency varies from six to 25 times per day. Treatment is very difficult since there is no effective therapy available to treat human cryptosporidiosis. Numerous drugs have been tried with no success. Supportive therapy in the form of anti-diarrhoeal drugs to manage the more serious diarrhoea and fluid replacement are required.

Table 9.1 summarizes the treatment of opportunistic infections in AIDS patients and emphasizes the difficulty in the management of these patients. Where effective therapy is available the patient usually shows an initial response but later may succumb to infection.

(2) TREATMENT OF KAPOSI'S SARCOMA

Local skin lesions (stages I and II) very rarely cause problems or need treatment but can be treated by surgical removal or by radiation

Table 9.2 Chemotherapy of AIDS-related Kaposi's sarcoma

Agent	Approximate objective response rate (complete + partial)
Vinblastine	40%
VP-16	75%
Adriamycin + bleomycin + vinblastine	75%
Alfa-Interferon	50%

therapy. For the more aggressive and disseminated form (stages III and IV) of Kaposi's sarcoma, chemotherapy with cytotoxic agents or interferon is the treatment of choice. A number of anticancer drugs have been employed including vinblastine, bleomycin, VP-16, and adriamycin (see Table 9.2). Although these are very active in the treatment of Kaposi's sarcoma unfortunately all of these types of drugs are very toxic and not selective for the tumour. They therefore may cause a further reduction in immune status since anticancer drugs usually attack actively dividing cells in the bone marrow and produce a fall in the production of white blood cells. Despite this major problem Kaposi's sarcoma does show some sensitivity to chemotherapy; however in many cases the lowered immune status whilst on chemotherapy gives rise to increased opportunistic infections which later kill the patient.

Interferon alfa in high doses has been used with some success to treat Kaposi's sarcoma and the interferons have the advantage that they do not suppress the immune system. Interferons are a family of biological substances that are produced naturally by animal cells in response to invasion by virus and some other agents. Interferons are anti-viral or viricidal and therefore help the body along with the immune system to cope with virus infections. The interferons have also been shown to be antiproliferative and so control the growth of some tumours. Furthermore since it is known that viruses can cause tumours in animals it seems that interferon is a likely candidate for the treatment of AIDS. Recently pure interferon has been made available in large quantities for clinical trial use. The method of production involves a relatively new technique called recombinant technology. In brief, human interferon is made by genetic engineering (or gene-splicing) whereby the human genetic material for interferon production is artificially introduced into a bacterial cell. The bacteria in culture then produce large amounts of interferon along with their other normal cellular components. Sophisticated purification processes then extract interferon from the culture medium. Interferons made by this recombinant process are usually of very high purity of around 98%.

In several clinical trials recombinant interferon has been demonstrated to be effective in the treatment of AIDS-related Kaposi's sarcoma. It also appears to be associated with a smaller incidence of life-threatening opportunistic infections when compared to other forms of chemotherapy. In several clinical studies throughout the United States, interferon has been shown to be of promise in the treatment of AIDS Kaposi's sarcoma, and in many centres alfa-interferon is the mainstay of therapy (see Table 9.2). However, along with other treatments, complete normalization of the immune deficiency has not been shown to occur and therefore the AIDS patient remains susceptible to opportunistic infections. Some interesting and exciting research has recently shown that interferon through its antiviral action is capable of suppressing the effects of HIV on lymphocytes. These studies suggest that clinical trials with interferon in early HIV infection are needed since it may be difficult to demonstrate significant antiviral effects in late disease.

An alternative therapeutic approach is to aim the treatment at the host rather than the tumour (Kaposi's sarcoma), that is, to correct the underlying immune deficiency.

(3) TREATMENT OF THE IMMUNE DEFICIENCY

At present there is no effective treatment for the underlying immune defect in AIDS. The presence of a cytopathic virus within the T-helper lymphocyte population makes attempts at treatment all the more difficult since it would be impossible to eliminate all virus from the patient.

A new development in recent years is the discovery of biological response modifiers which are able to modify the immune system. Many biological response modifying agents have been utilized in an effort to restore a balance in the immune status. Biological response modifying agents include:

- Interferon – alfa and gamma

- Interleukin II
- Thymic hormones (thymosin, thymopoietin)
- Mixed bacterial vaccine
- Monoclonal antibodies

Of the biological response modifiers only the interferons have so far shown any significant activity in AIDS.

(4) ANTI-HIV AGENTS – INHIBITORS OF VIRUS REPLICATION

One approach to effective antiviral therapy is to inhibit the viral enzyme reverse transcriptase which is responsible for viral replication in human cells. Reverse transcriptase enables the AIDS virus to convert RNA to DNA within the cell and start reproducing. The enzyme must be inhibited without interfering with the vital function of the helper T-cells. There are many compounds being investigated but the one that shows the most promise at present is azidothymidine (AZT). This inhibitor of reverse transcriptase has been shown to inhibit HIV replication in cell lines *in vitro* and shows promising results in studies to elucidate its potential in HIV infection in patients. AZT is also the first of the experimental drugs that can penetrate the brain where HIV often finds refuge.

Another reverse transcriptase inhibitor known as HPA-23 or antimoniotungstate is active against a broad spectrum of RNA and DNA viruses and has been tested in AIDS patients. The results so far have shown some activity for this drug in patients but toxicity has occurred and further studies are required.

It is not known if antiviral drugs are able to cure the disease since the virus (HIV) may have caused damage before treatment begins and the immune deficiency that results would be self-perpetuating even in the face of inhibition of HIV multiplication.

Antiviral agents:
- AZT (azidothymidine)
- Ribavirin
- Foscarnet (phosphonoformate)
- Suramin
- HPA 23 (antimoniotungstate)

Another antiviral agent and immunostimulant, inosine pranobex, has recently been made available for compassionate use in American and United Kingdom AIDS or PGL patients. The United States Food and Drug Administration (FDA) permitted use of inosine pranobex '... in a limited number of patients with PGL'. This move is believed to have resulted from the increasing concern of patients travelling to Mexico where the drug is available over the counter. A recent study in New York reported that treatment with inosine pranobex for 28 days was able to 'repair' the damaged immune system and might therefore help to prevent AIDS developing. Further studies are now under way in the United States, London and European countries to confirm the results of the New York study.

Alfa-interferon as previously mentioned may also be a useful antiviral drug and further work is in progress with this interesting agent.

Figure 9.1 summarizes the various strategies used in combating the AIDS virus.

A major difficulty that so far has occurred with all antiviral drugs is that HIV invariably returns after treatment is discontinued.

SUMMARY

The ideal drug for AIDS must:

(a) Stop the replication of HIV
(b) Permit regeneration of the immune system
(c) Be conveniently administered – preferably orally
(d) Be non-toxic over long periods – perhaps a lifetime
(e) Be active in the peripheral immune system cells and all other cells infected by HIV including the central nervous system.

So far no drug including AZT has been shown to meet these criteria.

(5) OTHER TREATMENT

(a) *Plasmapheresis*
Plasmapheresis is the removal of plasma from blood and reintroducing the cells into the patient. Its value has not yet been demonstrated in AIDS. Equipment is very expensive and only available at specialist centres.

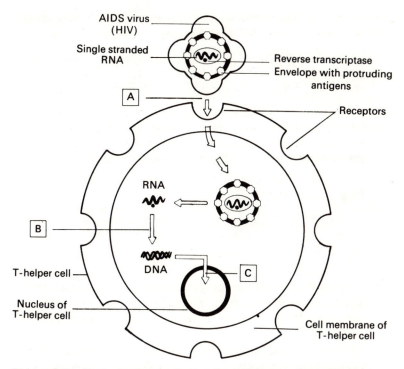

Figure 9.1 Strategies for combating the AIDS virus. **A:** within plasma: Neutralizing antibodies; **B:** within the T-cell: Inhibitors of reverse transcriptase; **C:** within T-cell nucleus: Inhibitors of viral replication

(b) *Bone marrow transplantation and leukocyte transfusion*
Bone marrow, the source of blood cells, is transplanted from a healthy donor into an AIDS patient. Transplants from identical twins may be beneficial and bone marrow transplantation merits further exploration in the treatment of AIDS. The biggest problem with this approach is that the replacement or graft bone marrow will eventually become infected.

(6) GENERAL MANAGEMENT AND PRECAUTIONS WHEN DEALING WITH AIDS PATIENTS

The Centers for Disease Control (CDC) in the United States have recommended the following precautions to hospitals and laboratories when dealing with AIDS patients:

(a) Extraordinary care must be taken to avoid accidental wounds from sharp instruments contaminated with potentially infectious material and to avoid contact of open skin lesions with material from AIDS patients.

(b) Gloves should be worn when handling blood specimens, blood-soiled items, body fluids, excretions, and secretions, as well as surfaces, materials, and objects exposed to them.

(c) Gowns should be worn when clothing may be soiled with body fluids, blood, secretions, or excretions.

(d) Hands should be washed after removing gowns and gloves and before leaving the rooms of known or suspected AIDS patients. Hands should also be washed thoroughly and immediately if they become contaminated with blood.

(e) Blood and other specimens should be labelled prominently with a special warning, such as 'Blood Precautions' or 'AIDS Precautions'. If the outside of the specimen container is visibly contaminated with blood, it should be cleaned with a disinfectant (such as a 1:10 dilution of 5.25% sodium hypochlorite (household bleach) with water). All blood specimens should be placed in a second container, such as an impervious bag, for transport. The container or bag should be examined for leaks or cracks.

(f) Blood spills should be cleaned up promptly with disinfectant solution, such as sodium hypochlorite (see above).

(g) Articles soiled with blood should be placed in an impervious bag prominently labelled 'AIDS Precautions' or 'Blood Precautions' before being sent for reprocessing or disposal. Alternatively, such contaminated items may be placed in plastic bags of a particular colour designated solely for disposal of infectious wastes by the hospital. Disposable items should be incinerated or disposed of in accord with the hospital's policies for disposal of infectious wastes. Reusable items should be reprocessed in accord with hospital policies for hepatitis B virus-contaminated items. Lensed instruments should be sterilized after use on AIDS patients.

(h) Needles should not be bent after use, but should be promptly placed in a puncture-resistant container used solely for such disposal. Needles should not be reinserted into their original sheaths before being discarded into the container, since this is a common cause of needle injury.

(i) Disposable syringes and needles are preferred. Only needle-locking syringes or one-piece needle-syringe units should be used to aspirate fluids from patients, so that collected fluid can be safely discharged through the needle, if desired. If reusable syringes are employed, they should be decontaminated before reprocessing.

(j) A private room is indicated for patients who are too ill to use good hygiene, such as those with profuse diarrhoea, faecal incontinence, or altered behaviour secondary to central nervous system infections.

In the United Kingdom the Association of Medical Microbiologists in collaboration with the Communicable Disease Surveillance Centre is mounting a surveillance programme to monitor exposed hospital workers. Anyone involved in the possible contamination of skin or mucosal surfaces (particularly 'needle stick' injuries) by the blood or body fluids of the patient with AIDS is asked to report the event to their local Infection Control Officer. A questionnaire will be sent out and a blood sample taken from the staff members to monitor for the appearance of HIV antibodies.

So far, in the United Kingdom there have been no cases of AIDS in health care workers including doctors, nurses, technicians, ancillary staff, except those in recognized high risk groups, for example homosexuals and intravenous drug users. Only one case – a nurse in England – has developed a positive antibody test to HIV from more than 500 health workers who have incurred needle stick injury and exposure to small amounts of blood from AIDS or at risk patients. It appears that AIDS represents considerably less risk than hepatitis B to health workers. Needle stick accidents are a frequent source of hepatitis B infection in medical personnel. A recent study has shown that the AIDS virus is not easily transmitted by prolonged close contact. None of a total of 101 physicians, nurses, technicians and other health workers at the San Francisco General Hospital who had prolonged close contacts with AIDS and ARC (AIDS-related complex) patients were found to have any evidence of infection with the virus associated with AIDS.

The mean period of exposure was 27 months; some of the most heavily exposed physicians and nurses had worked with AIDS patients for as long as 4 years. Exposures involved not only repeated 'hands-on' physical examinations and personal care but often splashes of blood or body fluids of AIDS patients. Sixteen persons had received needle sticks from AIDS or ARC patients; 4 had multiple needle sticks.

Despite such heavy exposures, a battery of tests for antibodies to the AIDS viruses failed to elicit a single instance of sero-conversion.

Dr Andrew Moss, and his colleagues at the University of California, San Francisco, who performed the research, emphasized that many of those studied had worked with AIDS patients before the disease was recognized and before the infection-control procedures for AIDS had been put in place. While AIDS transmission by needle stick and other occupational exposures must still be considered a possibility, they conclude, the likelihood of AIDS virus infection through casual contact is quite remote.

Laboratory investigations – British recommendations

If blood is taken from a person suspected of having AIDS or an HIV related condition then the following procedures outlined in the Advisory Committee on Dangerous Pathogens (ACDP) Guidelines issued by the DHSS (HC(85)2) should be observed:

(a) When blood or other specimens are to be taken, gloves and a disposable plastic apron and/or gown must be worn and discarded safely after use. Eye protection is recommended.

(b) Only the minimum essential quantity of blood should be drawn and then only by designated staff who are trained and experienced. Those who withdraw blood or other body fluids must ensure that the outside of any specimen container is free from contamination.

(c) Disposable units must be used for blood collection. Needles must be removed from syringes before the blood is discharged into the specimen container and immediately discarded into a puncture-proof disposable bin used solely for that purpose and designed for incineration. Only needle-locking syringes or similar units should be used to aspirate fluid from patients. Accidental puncture wounds in staff must be treated immediately by encouraging bleeding and liberal washing with soap and water. Any such accident or contamination of broken skin or mucous membranes must be promptly reported to and recorded by the person with overall responsibility for the work.

(d) Specimens must not be sent to the laboratory without a standing agreement between the clinician and senior laboratory staff. They must be in robust screw-capped and leak-proof containers (evacuated or not) bearing a hazard warning label. Securely capped specimen containers should be sent in separate sealed plastic bags, kept upright if possible and transported to the laboratory in a sound secondary container which can be disinfected. The accompanying request forms must be kept separate from the specimens to avoid contamination and also clearly indicate the hazard. Pins, staples or metal clips must not be used to seal the bags and for safety, the carrying handles of the secondary container should not be attached to the lid.

Chemical disinfectants that destroy HIV:

- Sodium hypochlorite (bleach) diluted 1 part bleach to 10 parts water
- Glutaraldehyde 2% freshly prepared
- 25% Ethanol

(7) COUNSELLING OF AIDS PATIENTS

(a) Taking Care of Yourself and Others

These guidelines have been adapted from the advice that the Terrence Higgins Trust gives to its counsellors who work with people with AIDS.

For further information on dealing with AIDS in the home contact the Terrence Higgins Trust on: 01–833 2971, 7 p.m.–10 p.m. Monday–Friday and 3 p.m.–10 p.m. at weekends.

If someone you know has AIDS it's important for you to know the simple precautions that you need to take to make your home safer for them and you – not that AIDS need be of any risk to you.

Remember that the AIDS virus has to enter directly into your blood stream in order to infect you.

Normal standard of household gloves will be enough to protect you from the germs that share your home. It makes good sense for EVERYONE – not just people with AIDS – to:

- Wash up in water and detergent hot enough to need gloves.
- Use different cleaning cloths for kitchen and bathroom.
- Make sure that meat is properly defrosted and cooked through.
- Wash your hands after handling pets or their litter trays.
- Wear gloves for gardening.
- If you cut yourself always put a sticking plaster or dressing over the wound.
- Toothbrushes, razors, sex toys should not be shared because of the risk of passing on small quantities of blood from one person to another.
- Guidelines for safer sex are given on page 119.

Blood, semen, vomit, and excrement are only dangerous when people don't know how to deal with them. Where possible these substances are best disposed of by the person who produced them. Spills of these substances should be wiped up and flushed away down the toilet. Then floors and surfaces affected can be disinfected by soaking for five minutes in diluted bleach – 1 part bleach to 10 parts water is recommended.

Dirty fabrics can be safely cleaned by using the hot water cycle in a washing machine. Modern fabrics might be damaged by a hot wash but it is far better to damage a fabric than to damage your health.

ALWAYS WEAR RUBBER GLOVES WHEN CLEANING UP SPILLS OF BODY FLUIDS.

(b) When a Friend has AIDS

This short list of suggestions has been put together by the counsellors of the Terrence Higgins Trust after working closely with people with AIDS.

Here are some thoughts and suggestions on ways to help your friend, lover, son, or anyone that you might know who has AIDS.

- A person with AIDS needs your friendship more than ever so it's important for him to know that you are a friend that he can trust and rely upon.

- Give him a hug or hold his hand, if you get the opportunity – he will enjoy the physical contact and the reassurance that goes with it. Remember some newspapers have tried to persuade him that he is a social leper.

- If he's on the phone, give him a call and gossip. If you intend to visit let him know about your intention to visit in advance. When someone is ill they tire easily so don't be offended if they don't want you to stay for long.

- Don't be afraid to show your emotions or to reveal how you feel. If you hold back your own thoughts and feelings a person who is ill will act in the same way. Remember he needs a friend who he can get close to and with whom he can relax and show how he really feels.

- Just because someone has AIDS doesn't mean that he wants to stay home all the time. If you have a car take him out for the day or evening. A visit to old haunts can be very therapeutic but be sure that you don't overtax him. If he's too ill for you to cope alone get a friend to help.

- He might find writing difficult either physically or emotionally so offer to help.

- If he wants to talk about his illness encourage him to do so. He may want to let off steam and you may be the ideal person on whom he can vent the anger or frustration he feels about being ill.

- If you have to go away for a short period or you can't visit try to keep in touch by phone or perhaps you could send a postcard.

- Just because someone is ill doesn't mean that he has lost interest in life. If he's gay make sure that he gets to see gay newspapers and magazines. Some of the national and local newspapers print a lot of rubbish about AIDS that will often upset someone with the illness. If you see something in the papers that might upset the people you know with AIDS then contact them and allow them the opportunity to talk it over with you.

● Try to keep up to date with what's happening medically to the person with AIDS and find out from the Terrence Higgins Trust about current medical research into AIDS. Hope is very important to someone with AIDS.

Table 9.3 Issues in AIDS-related counselling

Patients:
(1) Shock of diagnosis and facing possible death.
(2) Feeling of powerlessness to change circumstances, and consequent frustration and anger.
(3) Reduced physical functioning because of declining health.
(4) Anxiety about the reactions of others, with consequent social withdrawal and loss of social support.
(5) Reduced cognitive functioning because of anxiety, depression, obsessional worries, and possible intellectual impairment.
(6) Reduced sexual functioning, loss of libido, and erectile dysfunction.
(7) Fear of infecting others, particularly lovers, and fear of getting infection from them. .
(8) Concern about the lover, and how they can cope.
(9) Fear of being deserted and of dying alone.
(10) Fear of dying in pain and discomfort.
(11) Social, domestic, and occupational disruption.

Stable lovers:
(1) Fear about the possible death of the lover, grief, shock, and helplessness.
(2) Fear of becoming infected, leading to anxiety, depression, and obsessional worries.
(3) Reduced sexual functioning, especially loss of libido and loss of prospect of future sex.
(4) Guilt about the possibility of having infected the partner and others.
(5) Uncertainty about what to do next; conflict between avoiding infection and love of the partner; guilt about this conflict.
(6) Uncertainty about what to do to help the partner.
(7) Clinical anxiety and depression.

Contacts, PGL patients, and those fearing AIDS:
(1) Anxiety about having AIDS or the virus.
(2) Depression about the perceived inevitability of infection, and/or developing the full syndrome.
(3) Morbid obsession about the disease with ruminations and checking for symptoms.
(4) Guilt about being homosexual and the resurrection of past 'misdemeanours'.
(5) Social, domestic, and occupational disruption and stress.

Table reproduced from David Miller and John Green

Table 9.4   Guidelines for safer sex

Patients:
  (1) Maintain sexual activity **only** with established stable partner.
  (2) **Inform** established partner of the necessity for fidelity.
  (3) **No** anal intercourse (active or passive).
  (4) **No** oral–anal sex.
  (5) **No** oral–genital sex or exposure to partner's urine.
  (6) **No** 'wet' kissing.
  (7) Keep **only** to mutual masturbation, body-rubbing, and 'dry' kissing.

Stable lovers:
  (1) **No** anal intercourse (active or passive).
  (2) **No** oral–anal sex.
  (3) **No** oral–genital sex or exposure to partner's urine.
  (4) **No** 'wet' kissing.
  (5) **No** new partners.
  (6) Keep **only** to (mutual) masturbation, body-rubbing, and 'dry' kissing.
  (7) **Regular** venereological screenings and prompt treatment of infections.

Contacts, virus-infected, and PGL patients:
  (1) **Restrict** sex to known (preferably only one existing) partner.
  (2) **No** anal sex (active or passive).
  (3) **No** oral–anal sex.
  (4) **No** oral–genital sex, or exposure to partner's urine.
  (5) **No** 'wet' kissing.
  (6) Keep **only** to (mutual) masturbation, body-rubbing, and 'dry' kissing.
  (7) **No** new partners.
  (8) **Regular** venereological screenings and prompt treatment of infections.

Others:
  (1) **Restrict** sex to known (preferably one only) partner, or to a closed circle of contacts.
  (2) **No** anal intercourse (active or passive).
  (3) **No** oral–anal or oral–genital sex, or exposure to urine.
  (4) **No** 'wet' kissing.
  (5) Keep **only** to (mutual) masturbation, body-rubbing, and 'dry' kissing.
  (6) **No** sex with people from high-risk areas (America, Africa, Haiti).
  (7) **Prompt** treatment of venereological infections.

Table reproduced from David Miller and John Green

Guidelines for Safe Sex Activities

Low risk/fairly safe
● mutual and group masturbation
● 'dry' kissing (no exchange of saliva)
● sex toys (dildos, vibrators, butt plugs, *etc*) used with partner but not shared

- bondage, beating, whipping and spanking as long as skin is not broken
- body-to-body contact
- penis-to-body contact, except between thighs and buttocks

Medium risk
- 'wet' kissing (with exchange of saliva)
- coitus interfemoris (penis-to-body contact between thighs or buttocks)
- fingering (putting fingers into the anus)
- douches and enemas
- fellatio (swallowing semen may not increase risk)
- cunnilingus
- urination (water sports) as long as the urine does not enter the mouth, anus or eyes

Higher risk
- sharing sex toys
- anilingus (rimming or tonguing)
- brachoproctic stimulation (fisting – putting the hand, fist or forearm into the rectum)

Highest risk
- vaginal sex ⎫ may be safer if condom used
- anal sex ⎭ (use a water-based lubricant)
- any sex act that draws blood
- enemas and douches before and after anal sex

Safe sex – AIDS and the condom

Since HIV is transmitted primarily through blood, seminal fluid and female genital secretions any barrier to these fluids should reduce disease transmission. This has formed the basis of safe sex guidelines that using condoms confers some protection against AIDS.

There is reasonable but not exhaustive evidence that condoms confer protection. Certainly HIV is unable to pass through the latex of condoms and a recent study has shown a decrease in the spread of HIV in adults with AIDS who used condoms on a regular basis. There is good evidence that condoms prevent the spread of other sexually transmitted diseases.

Current use of condoms is spread unevenly through the world. Japan accounts for about 27% of all condom users (the oral contraceptive pill is rarely used), 38% in the rest of the developed world, 18% in China, Latin America and the Caribbean account for only 3% of world condom use. Africa and the Middle East account for only 1%.

Modern condoms may not be strong enough when used for anal sex but tougher sheaths are available and are used by homosexual men particularly in North America. Preliminary evidence appears to show that the 'safe sex' campaign is working. In San Francisco the annual rate at which gay men were becoming HIV-positive has fallen from 17% in 1982–84 to 4% in 1984–85, while the incidence of rectal gonorrhoea has fallen by 71% between 1983 and 1985.

In London in mid-1986, 77% of gay men questioned claimed to follow 'safe-sex' guidelines. The city's incidence of sexually transmitted diseases among homosexual men has fallen.

Other barrier methods such as the cap, diaphragm or sponges offer some protection against HIV transmission but are not thought to be as effective as condoms.

CHAPTER 10

Endpiece

AIDS is a frightening disease since it has dire consequences for its victims. The prevalence of AIDS appears to be increasing at an alarming rate. Epidemiologists and other scientific researchers are trying to track the spread of the disease and define more accurately the various risk factors involved in the development of AIDS. At the present time it is thought that between 30 000 to 100 000 in the United Kingdom and 1 million to 1.5 million people in the United States are infected with HIV. If all of these go on to develop AIDS then clearly there will exist a serious and devastating health problem.

Forecasting the number of people with AIDS is compounded with difficulties – the most difficult of which is the uncertainty concerning the future spread of the virus. Another major factor is the percentage of infected patients who go on to develop AIDS. Leading specialists have stated that anything from 10% to 100% of HIV infected individuals will eventually develop AIDS. Assuming 50% of carriers develop AIDS by 1992 in the UK there could be an accumulative total of 20 000 to 50 000 cases of AIDS, of whom about half would have died.

A further estimate suggests that up to 20 000 individuals in the UK could be infected by HIV by 1988 with over 3000 cases of AIDS. In the United States forecasts suggest that the total number of cases of AIDS in 1991 will be around 270 000.

A major research effort is under way in many countries including the United States, France and the United Kingdom which has produced a plethora of data on AIDS. However we still do not fully understand the factors involved in the course of the disease. We know even less about how to treat this serious disorder.

New cases of AIDS appear daily and our ideas on the epidemiology, cause and management of AIDS patients and patients at risk will change with time. Even within a matter of a few months our knowledge of this disorder will greatly increase and what we know and do today will be history tomorrow.

Glossary

AIDS

Acquired immune deficiency syndrome.

AIDS-related complex (ARC)

A variety of chronic symptoms and signs that occur in some persons infected with HIV but whose condition does not meet the definition of AIDS. About 50% of patients with ARC go on to develop AIDS.

aetiology

The study of the cause of a disease.

allergen

An antigen that causes an allergic reaction.

anaemia

Condition in which there is a reduction in number of circulating red blood cells or in haemoglobin. Clinically, anaemia is manifested by pallor, shortness of breath, palpitations and fatigue.

antibody

Protein secreted by plasma cells (activated B-cells) which interacts with a specific antigen to neutralize it, forming an antigen–antibody complex.

antibody test

Measuring specific antibodies to infection with HIV in the laboratory detects evidence of HIV in the blood.

antigen
A class of substances that stimulate production of antibodies. Specific antigens protruding from the cell membrane, the so-called cell surface 'markers', help the body to identify the cell.

antiproliferative
A substance that stops cellular reproduction. Usually refers to substances that prevent the reproduction of cancer cells. Normal body cells may also be affected, for example the bone marrow and intestines.

antiviral agent
A substance that prevents or treats a viral infection.

autoimmune disease
Disease in which the body produces an immunological response directed against own body.

axilla
The armpit.

biopsy
The surgical removal of a piece of tissue for examination under a microscope.

bleomycin
An antitumour antibiotic.

B-lymphocyte (B-cell)
Lymphocyte derived from bone marrow stem cells that, upon stimulation by a specific antigen, becomes a plasma cell and secretes antibodies against the antigen.

bone marrow
Spongy tissue in the middle of bones that produces blood cells.

bronchoscopy
Examination of the bronchi through a fibre-optic instrument (bronchoscope).

cancer
A malignant tumour; a mass or swelling resulting from uncontrolled cell division.

cancer chemotherapy
The practice of administering one or more anti-cancer drugs to reduce the tumour burden.

carcinogen
A substance that can cause or help cause cancer.

carcinoma
A cancer that develops from epithelial cells. These cells are present in the skin, lungs, glands, gastrointestinal tract, and urinary tract. Cancers that develop in these sites are called carcinomas and are the commonest type of cancer.

cell-mediated immunity
That part of the immune system in which T-cells become activated, multiply and secrete lymphokines when stimulated by a specific antigen.

chromosome
The chromosome consists of DNA and carries the genes or factors of inheritance.

combination chemotherapy
Administering two or more anti-cancer agents together in an attempt to reduce the tumour burden or achieve a cure. Drug combinations are usually chosen to exert a prolonged and synergistic action.

computerized tomography (CT)
Special radiographing (X-ray) of a selected level of the body utilizing a computer.

connective tissue
General supporting or connecting tissue of the body formed of elongated flattened cells held together by a loose network of non-cellular fibres.

cytotoxic drug
In oncology, an agent that inhibits or prevents the function of the cell, thus interfering with cell division.

differentiation
A maturation process by which cells of identical genetic make-up become structurally and functionally different from one another,

according to the genetically controlled development programme of the species.

DNA (deoxyribonucleic acid)
The hereditary material of the cell – nucleic acid found in the nucleus that carries the genetic information for all living cells, transmitting it from one generation to the next.

ELISA
An acronym for 'enzyme-linked immunosorbent assay' a test used to detect antibodies against HIV.

encephalitis
Inflammation of the brain.

encephalopathy
A degenerative disease of the brain.

endemic
Said of a disease continually present in a particular region or community.

endothelium
Layer of flat cells lining the body cavities, the inside surface of the digestive tube (intestine) and other organs, blood vessels and lymph vessels.

epidemic
A disease attacking a large number of people in a community simultaneously.

epidemiology
The study of the prevalence and spread of a disease in a community.

erythrocyte
The mature erythrocyte or red blood cell which has no nucleus. The erythrocyte carries oxygen, bound to haemoglobin, to the cells of the body.

false negative
Denotes a test result that wrongly excludes an individual from a diagnostic or other category.

false positive
Denotes a test result that wrongly assigns an individual to a diagnostic or other category.

gene
The biological unit of heredity located on chromosomes and made of DNA. Each gene is located at a definite position on a particular chromosome. (A virus has about 100 genes; man about 150 000.)

granulocyte
Leukocyte (white blood cell) whose cytoplasm contains granules (small specks of membrane-enclosed enzymes). Granulocytes are produced in the bone marrow and constitute the body's first line of defence.

haemophilia
hereditary bleeding disorder caused by a deficiency of a blood clotting factor.

helper T-cells
A type of T-lymphocyte that helps control the responses of both cytotoxic T-cells and antibody producing B-cells during a specific immune response.

histology/histopathology
The study of tissues and diseased tissue under the microscope.

human immunodeficiency virus (HIV)
The causative agent of AIDS.

humoral immunity
That part of the specific immune response in which the B-cells, when activated by an antigen, become plasma cells and secrete antibody.

hypersensitivity reactions
An exaggerated and inappropriate immune reaction, usually against a foreign antigen that causes damage to body tissues or exerts other effects.

immune complex
Antibody and antigen combined together.

immune deficiency
A state, inherited or acquired, in which the immune system is deficient.

immune system
The body defence system that fights against invasion by bacteria, viruses, fungi, parasites, malignant cells and other substances that are recognized by the body as 'non-self'. It includes white blood cells called phagocytes (granulocytes, monocytes) that engulf the invaders, lymphocytes (B-cells, plasma cells) that produce antibodies to neutralize the invaders, and lymphocytes (T-cells) that kill invaders by direct contact.

immunocompetence
The ability to respond immunologically to antigens.

immunoglobulin
An antibody; one of a class of proteins that interact specifically with antigens. Produced by B-cells and plasma cells.

immunomodulation
Process that alters the activity of one or more of the components of the immune system.

immunomodulators
Class of agents produced which stimulate cell action.

immunosuppression
Suppression of the body's normal immune defence systems.

immunotherapy
An experimental method of treatment that attempts to increase the body's own defence (immune) mechanisms.

incidence
The rate at which a certain event occurs, such as the number of new cases of AIDS occurring during a certain period.

inflammation
A reaction in the tissues characterized by redness, swelling and pain. It is a consequence of many local immune reactions.

interferons
Family of natural proteins produced locally by certain nucleated cells of vertebrates (humans, monkeys, chickens, etc.) when they are attacked by a virus. They exert a non-specific, early defence against viral infection. Interferons possess antiviral, antiproliferative and immunomodulatory activity.

There are three classes of interferons, each with further subclasses:

Alfa-interferon – the interferon secreted by white blood cells (leukocytes). There are over 14 subclasses of human alfa-interferon.

Beta-interferon – the interferon secreted by fibroblasts (connective tissue cells).

Gamma-interferon – secreted by T-cells following exposure to antigen. Acts as a lymphokine, stimulates monocytes and macrophages as well as other cells.

interleukin
A molecule secreted by a white blood cell which transmits a signal to another white blood cell.

Kaposi's sarcoma
A malignant tumour made up of cells that resemble embryonic connective tissue. It principally involves the skin, although other organs such as the intestines may be affected. Characterized by reddish blue or brownish skin nodules.

killer (K) cell
A cell of the immune system (lymphocyte) that destroys virus infected cells once they are coated with antibody.

lentiviruses
A subfamily of retroviruses that includes the visna viruses of sheep and the infectious anaemia virus of horses, that cause chronic diseases in their natural hosts. Researchers believe that HIV belongs to the lentivirus subfamily.

leukocyte
White blood cell. Leukocytes are divided into two major groups: (1) granulocytes, originating in the bone marrow and involved in non-specific body defence; (2) lymphocytes, originating in the bone marrow (B-cells) or lymphatic tissues (T-cells) and participating in the immune defence of the body.

localized cancer
A cancer confined to the site of origin.

lymph
A clear, colourless fluid that flows through the lymphoid system.

lymph node
Small oval or bean shaped bodies of various sizes found along the course of a lymphatic vessel. It is composed chiefly of lymphocytes and connective tissue.

lymphadenopathy
Swollen lymph glands in part or throughout the body.

lymphatic system
Circulatory network of lymph-carrying vessels, the lymph nodes, spleen, and thymus that functions as a place for the production, storage and immune activities of the lymphocytes.

lymphocyte
A cell of the immune system that gives rise to T-cells, B-cells, Killer (K) cells and Natural Killer (NK) cells which participate in the specific immune response.

lymphoma
A term applied to a malignant disease of lymphoid tissue and includes Burkitt's lymphoma and Hodgkin's lymphoma.

lysis
Dissolution or breakdown of the cell.

macrophage
Large scavenger cells fixed in the lining of organs such as the liver and lungs. Macrophages are thought to originate from monocytes (a type of white blood cell) that become immobilized in certain tissues.

malignant transformation
Alteration in a normal cell's characteristics to make it into a cancer cell.

memory (immunological)
The phenomenon in which a secondary encounter with the same antigen produces a more vigorous immune response than that which followed the initial exposure to antigen. Memory is carried by lymphocytes previously exposed to specific antigen.

memory cells
Specific lymphocytes primed by contact with antigen that react more rapidly upon second contact with the same antigen. The memory cells may persist for many years.

messenger RNA (mRNA)
A nucleic acid that transcribes a coded genetic message from a region of DNA and carries it to a ribosome, where it serves as the template for protein synthesis. Abbreviated as mRNA.

metastasis
The spread of a cancer from one part of the body to another. The new area of cancer is a metastasis or secondary.

monocyte
Large leukocytes (white blood cells) originating from the same primitive (stem) cell as the granulocyte in the bone marrow, but having distinct functions. Monocytes are mobile scavengers that kill cells recognized as 'non-self' without prior exposure (non-specific cell-mediated immunity).

mortality rate
The death rate.

myelosuppression
Suppression of normal bone marrow function leading to a diminished production of red blood cells and white blood cells. May be associated with anaemia, thrombocytopenia, leukopenia.

natural killer (NK) cell
A lymphocyte that specifically attacks virally infected and cancer cells and releases interferon upon activation.

neoplasm
Literally means 'new tissue' or 'new growth'. The growth may be malignant or benign.

neutrophils
Infection fighting white blood cells. Also called polymorpho-nuclear neutrophils.

neutralizing antibodies
An antibody which when mixed with the specific antigen reduces the amount of antigen and renders it neutral.

nucleic acid
Two types of nucleic acid occur in nature: deoxyribonucleic acid (DNA) and ribonucleic acid (RNA). Nucleic acid is made up of long chains of building blocks called nucleotides of which four types each make up DNA and RNA.

nucleus
The central point of the cell that houses the hereditary information, deoxyribonucleic acid – DNA.

oncogenic
Giving rise to cancer.

oncology
Study of cancer and its treatment.

organelle
A specialized functional unit (for example, the nucleus) embedded within the cytoplasm of a cell.

pathology
The branch of medicine concerned with the examination of diseased tissues.

phagocytosis
The engulfing behaviour of certain white blood cells.

plasma cell
A short-lived derivative of a B-lymphocyte that has been activated by an antigen and secretes antibodies.

preclinical
Refers to *in vitro* and *in vivo* studies performed in animals.

premalignant
An abnormal area that shows changes that may lead to malignancy but has not, as yet, done so.

prevalence
The number of cases of a disease present in a specified population at a given time.

prognosis
A prediction of the likely course of a disease. This can only be estimated from the experiences of a lot of patients and cannot accurately predict the outcome in an individual.

prophylactic
Treatment designed to prevent a disease.

protein
Proteins serve as enzymes, hormones, immunoglobulins and form

the principal constituents of protoplasm. Each protein has a unique, genetically determined amino acid sequence which determines its specific shape and function.

radiation therapy
Administration of ionizing radiation to kill cancerous cells.

relapse (recurrence) of cancer
The regrowth of a cancer after it has been removed or has responded to treatment.

replication
The process of duplicating or reproducing, as the replication of an exact copy of a strand of viral DNA or RNA. The process by which a chromosome forms a copy of itself.

retrovirus
RNA viruses that have an enzyme (reverse transcriptase) that can cause a DNA copy of the viral RNA to be made. Retroviruses cause sarcomas and leukaemias in animals as well as leukaemias and AIDS in humans.

serology
The scientific study of serum.

seronegative
A condition in which no antibodies can be detected to a particular organism.

seropositive
A condition in which antibodies to a particular organism are found in the blood. Indicates that the individual has been exposed to the organism.

serum
The clear liquid that separates from blood when it is allowed to clot.

skin test
The injection of small amounts of specific antigen into the skin to cause a local immune response indicative of a hypersensitivity reaction.

spleen
Large, elongated lymphoid organ in the upper left abdomen. It also functions as a trap for aged and damaged red cells.

staging of tumour
The systemic investigation of the extent of spread of tumour. The amount of tumour spread is described as the disease stage.

stem cell
An immature cell, which through repeated replication, gives rise to mature cells with a commitment to a specific function.

suppressor T-cell
A type of T-lymphocyte that releases special substances called lymphokines that stop antibody production by plasma cells and B-cells.

supraclavicular
The area above the clavicle (collar bone). May refer to lymph nodes at this site.

survival time
Length of time a patient can be expected to live given a particular disease.

systemic
Refers to the whole body, hence systemic treatment treats the whole body.

T-cell
A lymphocyte cell derived from the thymus gland that participates in a variety of cell-mediated immune reactions. Subsets of T-cells have a variety of specialized functions in the immune system (see helper T-cells and suppressor T-cells).

thymus gland
Important in maintaining cellular immunity in that T-cells reach maturity in this organ. The thymus may be removed or destroyed in experimental animals to induce immunodeficiency.

tolerance
The state of immunological unresponsiveness, as is normally the case with respect to the body's own tissues.

transformed cell
A cancer cell.

transfusion
The introduction of blood or blood products directly into the blood stream.

tumour
A growth arising from normal tissue, but independent of the normal rate of growth of such a tissue and serves no physiological function. Literally means a swelling or mass.

tumour burden
Estimate of the total number of cancer cells present in the patient's body.

vaccination
The intentional exposure of the body to an antigen in such a way that it generates specific acquired immunity against that antigen.

vinblastine
Anticancer agent derived from the periwinkle plant.

viraemia
Presence of viruses in the bloodstream. Causes symptoms such as chills, fever etc.

viral interference
Phenomenon observed in which the presence of a viral infection prevents infection by a second virus. This observation led to the discovery of interferon.

virus
A group of minute infectious agents not discernible by light microscopy (in contrast to bacteria). It is one of the smallest infectious particles known. It lacks an independent metabolism so it can replicate (reproduce) only within a living host cell. Thus it is sometimes called an intracellular parasite. The virus particle, or virion, contains only one kind of nucleic acid DNA or RNA contained within a protein shell.

VP-16 (etoposide)
Anticancer extract of the May apple that shows activity in the treatment of Kaposi's sarcoma.

Western blot technique
A test that involves the identification of antibodies against specific protein molecules. The test is more specific than ELISA in detecting HIV antibodies in blood samples and is often used as a confirmatory test on samples found to be repeatedly positive in the ELISA test.

AIDS – Important information for blood donors

AIDS is short for Acquired Immune Deficiency Syndrome. It is a very serious disease caused by a virus which depresses the body's resistance to infections and other illnesses. It is not transmitted by ordinary day-to-day social contact.

HOW IS AIDS TRANSMITTED?

The transmission of AIDS is not yet fully understood, but it is known that one means of transmitting the disease is through blood and blood products. Because of this, all blood donations are now being tested for antibody to the AIDS virus, but people in the groups most likely to be at risk from AIDS still MUST NOT GIVE BLOOD.

WHO IS MOST AT RISK FROM AIDS?

The high risk groups are:

(1) Homosexual and bisexual men.
(2) Drug abusers, both men and women, who inject drugs.
(3) Haemophiliacs who have been treated with blood products.
(4) Sexual contacts of people in these groups.

HOW CAN THE RISKS TO OTHERS BE REDUCED?

People in the high risk groups MUST NOT GIVE BLOOD. They should not attend donor sessions. The test may not pick up early cases of infection.

WHERE CAN THOSE AT RISK BE TESTED?

People in the high risk groups can be tested either through their own doctor or a Sexually Transmitted Diseases (STD) clinic – in the strictest confidence.

HOW WILL BLOOD DONATIONS BE TESTED?

Occasionally donors may unknowingly carry the AIDS virus in their bodies. A test for anaemia is made before donation. Further tests for certain diseases are done later in the laboratory and these will now include the test for antibody to the AIDS virus. Donors will be asked to agree to the test.

HOW ARE THE RESULTS NOTIFIED?

In the very unlikely event of any of these tests being positive, a donor will be informed by the Regional Transfusion Director so that additional confirmatory tests can be arranged. A donor's medical history is always kept in the strictest confidence.

CAN DONORS GET AIDS BY GIVING BLOOD?

Absolutely not. Neither AIDS nor any other disease can be contracted from giving blood. All the materials used for collecting blood are sterile and are used only once.

Donors can discuss in confidence whether to give blood

- with a doctor at the blood collection session
- with their own doctor
- with the Director of their Blood Transfusion Centre
- at any Sexually Transmitted Diseases (STD) clinic.

To find your nearest clinic look in the phone book under Venereal Diseases.

REMEMBER, AIDS IS A SERIOUS DISEASE

Please do **not** give blood

- if you are a homosexual or bisexual man
- if you are a drug abuser who injects drugs
- if you are a haemophiliac who has been treated with blood products
- if you are a sexual contact of any of these people.

Our concern is for your safety and the safety of the patient who receives your blood.

Acquired Immune Deficiency Syndrome AIDS

WHO Consultation

An international conference on AIDS, sponsored by the United States Department of Health and Human Services and the World Health Organization, was held in Atlanta, Georgia (United States of America), on 15–17 April 1985. It was attended by over 2000 participants from 50 countries, and was followed on 18–19 April by a WHO consultation to review the information presented at the conference and to assess its international implications. The group of consultants concluded that the information available today is sufficient to permit health authorities to take action which may reduce the incidence of AIDS among certain risk groups.

Following are the main conclusions and recommendations of the consultation:

For WHO:

• Establish a network of collaborating centres with special expertise in the field. The centres should assist in the training of staff, the provision of reference panels of sera and the evaluation of diagnostic tests, as well as advise on the production of working reagents. They should also assist in the preparation of educational material and the organization of studies to determine the natural history of the diseases and the extent of infection in different parts of the world.

- Coordinate the global surveillance of AIDS using a compatible reporting format and the currently accepted case definition. The Organization should disseminate this data as well as new information on the disease as widely and rapidly as possible.

- Assist in the development of an effective vaccine and, when appropriate, in the establishment of international requirements for the vaccine. WHO should play an active role in facilitating the evaluation of candidate vaccines.

For Member States:

- The public should be informed that HIV infection is acquired through heterosexual and homosexual intercourse, needle-sharing by intravenous drug users, transfusion of contaminated blood and blood products, transmission by infected mothers to their babies, and probably through repeated use of needles and other unsterile instruments used for skin piercing. Information should be provided about the risk of HIV infection and AIDS, especially to those persons, both men and women, who may be at increased risk because of multiple sexual partners. There is currently no evidence of the spread of HIV by casual social contact, or within households. Countries which have yet to recognize AIDS should know that provision of timely and accurate information on this point is often necessary to allay inappropriate public concern.

- Countries should ensure that health care workers are informed about AIDS and HIV infection, modes of transmission, clinical spectrum, available programme of management including psychosocial support, and methods for prevention and control.

- Each country should assess the risk that AIDS poses to its population and establish methods of diagnosis through surveillance and laboratory testing, including specific tests for HIV.

- Since HIV infection precedes AIDS in an individual or a community, early recognition will require serological studies in groups with potential risk of infection. WHO should encourage and assist in periodic serological studies in countries where AIDS has yet to be recognized and should ensure the collection of comparable data and a representative selection of sera.

- Where feasible, potential donors of blood and plasma should be screened for antibody to HIV, and positive units should not be used for either the transfusion or the manufacture of products where there is a risk of transmitting infectious agents. Potential donors should be informed about the testing in advance of the donation.

- Risks of transmission of HIV by Factor VIII and IX concentrates can be reduced through treatment by heat or other proven methods of inactivation. The use of such products is recommended.

- Potential donors of organs, sperms, or other human material should be informed about AIDS and groups at increased risk of infection should exclude themselves from donating. Whenever possible serological testing should be performed before these materials are used. This is particularly important when donor material is collected from an unconscious or deceased patient on whom relevant information may be lacking.

- Individuals with positive tests for antibody HIV should be referred for medical evaluation and counselling. Such people should inform their health care attendants of their status.

- Health authorities should develop guidelines for the total care of patients and handling of their specimens in hospitals and other settings. These guidelines should be similar to those which have been effective for care of patients with hepatitis B.

- Countries are strongly advised to develop codes of good laboratory practice to protect staff against the risk of infection. Such recommendations may be based upon those found in the Laboratory Biosafety Manual published by WHO in 1983. The level of care required for work with specimens from patients infected with HIV is similar to that required with hepatitis B. The use of class II biological safety cabinets is recommended. These cabinets are adequate for containment of other agents such as herpes and hepatitis viruses, mycobacteria, and protozoa which may be present in the specimens. For work involving production and purification of HIV, biosafety containment level 3 (P-3) must be employed.

- The collection and storage of serum samples from representative laboratory workers at the time of employment and at regular intervals thereafter is encouraged to assess the risk of laboratory-acquired infection and the effectiveness of biosafety guidelines. Countries should provide this information to WHO for correlation and dissemination. Provision of samples and testing should be carried out with the informed consent of the subjects.

- Countries should be aware of the importance of confidentiality of information about the results of serological testing and the identity of AIDS patients. Serological testing should be undertaken with the informed consent of the subject.

APPENDIX 4

Cellular immunity

LYMPHOCYTES

Lymphocytes are white blood cells which originate in the bone marrow but also reside in the lymphatic system. The lymphatic system is a continuous series of ducts and nodes (lymph glands) carrying lymph which is rather like blood plasma. Two lymphocyte sub-populations have a specific role in the immune system: B-cells and T-cells.

(1) B-cells (B-lymphocytes) are named after the bursa, an organ in birds where cells with similar function were first observed. In response to antigen (a foreign particle), B-cells synthesize antibody. The antigen–antibody complex which is formed renders the antigen inactive and it can then be removed by other cells called phagocytes. Once a B-cell has learned to synthesize an antibody, it divides and multiplies forming a clone of cells, all capable of producing the same antibody. If the same antigen reappears at a later date a whole clone of B-cells is available to produce antibody specifically against the antigen (see Figure A4.1).

(2) T-cells (T-lymphocytes) are thought to be processed by the thymus gland, a gland in the upper chest just below the neck.

There are about eight or nine subsets of T-cells that so far have been identified. However, two of these are particularly relevant to our discussion of AIDS:

(a) Helper cells – These help other immune defence cells such as

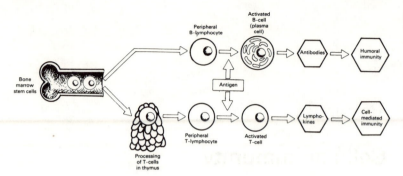

Figure A4.1   The formation and functions of lymphocytes

the antibody producing B-lymphocytes, to act against foreign invaders.

(b) Suppressor cells – These decrease the activity of immune defence cells.

The normal ratio between helper to suppressor cells is about 2.4:1. i.e. about twice as many helper cells as suppressor cells. In AIDS patients the ratio may be reversed – there are more suppressor than helper cells, that is the number of T-helper cells is markedly reduced. This is thought to be attributable to a depletion of T-helper cells. This acquired depression or depletion of T-helper cells is the hallmark of fully-expressed AIDS. HIV is 'lymphotropic' for T-helper cells; the virus replicates within these cells and destroys them thus bringing damage to the immune system.

The laboratory test for lymphocyte subsets is available only in certain specialized centres.

In AIDS the defect in cellular immunity leads to infection with opportunistic agents particularly viruses, protozoa and fungi. The immune deficiency also leads to the development of tumours, particularly Kaposi's sarcoma and lymphomas.

There are also many other cellular immune abnormalities that have been described in AIDS and in pre-AIDS. This is a complex subject and outside the remit of this discussion, but interested readers are referred to the selected bibliography for further reading. A brief discussion follows:

Table A4.1   Immunological abnormalities in AIDS

A. *Characteristic pattern*
  (1) Quantitative T-lymphocyte deficiency
    ● Total T-lymphocytopenia
    ● Selective T-helper lymphocytopenia

  (2) Qualitative T-lymphocyte defect
    ● Functional defect
    ● Selective functional defect of T-helper subset

  (3) Hyperactivity of B-cell response
    ● Increased spontaneous immunoglobulin secretion by B-cells
    ● Elevated serum immunoglobulin levels

B. *Consistently observed pattern (probably secondary to A)*
  (1) Decreased *in vitro* lymphocyte proliferative responses

  (2) Decreased cytotoxic responses
    ● Natural killer cells
    ● Cell-mediated cytotoxicity (T-cell)

  (3) Altered monocyte function.

C. *Other reported abnormalities*
  (1) Increased levels of acid labile interferon

  (2) Anti-lymphocyte antibodies

  (3) Increased levels of β_2-microglobulin and α_1-thymosin

IMMUNOLOGICAL ABNORMALITIES IN AIDS

The immunological abnormalities in AIDS are sweeping. The common denominator of the immune defects in AIDS is a quantitative and qualitative defect in T-helper cells, leading to a profound defect in cell-mediated immunity (see Table A4.1).

The original observations on the immunological defects in AIDS indicated that the defect was only at a level of the T-cell limb of the immune response. However, AIDS patients also show an abnormality of B-cell function characterized by a polyclonal activation of B-cells with spontaneous secretion of immunoglobulin. This may explain the hypergammaglobulinaemia which is consistently seen in AIDS patients. Therefore, the presence of hypergammaglobulinaemia does not indicate an intact B-cell limb, but rather a hyperactive B-cell repertoire. Recent evidence has shown that HIV may also infect

B-cell lines and some monocytes and this may explain the B-cell abnormalities seen in AIDS.

AIDS patients also manifest defects in T-cell and natural killer (NK) cell-mediated cytotoxicity. Monocyte function is also abnormal in AIDS (see Table A4.1 for details).

There are many other reported immunological abnormalities in AIDS patients (e.g. increased levels of acid labile alfa-interferon) but their clinical significance has not been elucidated.

Definition and revision of the case definition of AIDS used by Centers for Disease Control (CDC) Atlanta, USA, June 1985. Case definition of AIDS in children

DEFINITION OF AIDS

The original case definition for AIDS established by the Centers for Disease Control in the United States and subsequently adopted by the World Health Organisation and national health authorities including those in the UK was:

(i) A reliably diagnosed disease that is at least moderately indicative of an underlying cellular immune deficiency. For example, Kaposi's sarcoma in a patient aged less than 60 years, or opportunistic infection.

(ii) No known underlying cause of the cellular immune deficiency nor any other cause of reduced resistance reported to be associated with the disease.

Table A5.1 lists those diseases at least moderately indicative of underlying cellular immune deficiency.

In June 1985, this definition was revised following the discovery of the causative agent and in recognition of the wider range of clinical manifestations experience had shown to be associated with HIV.

Table A5.1 Diseases indicative of underlying cellular
immunodeficiency

Protozoal and helminthic

Cryptosporidiosis ⎫
Isosporiasis ⎬ Diarrhoea for >1 month
Pneumocystis carinii pneumonia

Strongyloidosis — Pneumonia, CNS, or disseminated
Toxoplasmosis — Pneumonia or CNS

Fungal
Aspergillosis — CNS or disseminated
Candidiasis — Oesophageal or
bronchopulmonary
Cryptococosis — Pulmonary, CNS, or disseminated
Histoplasmosis — Disseminated

Bacterial
'Atypical' mycobacteriosis — (Species other than tuberculosis
or lepra) disseminated

Viral
Cytomegalovirus — Pulmonary, gut or CNS
Herpes simplex virus — Severe mucocutaneous disease
>1 month, pulmonary, gut or
disseminated

Progressive multifocal
leukoencephalopathy

Cancer
Kaposi's sarcoma — No age restriction
Cerebral lymphoma
Non-Hodgkin's lymphoma — Diffuse, undifferentiated, and of
B-cell or unknown phenotype
Lymphoreticular malignancy — >3 months after an opportunistic
infection

Other
Chronic lymphoid interstitial
pneumonitis in child under 13
years

Patients suffering such illnesses but showing negative results on testing for
antibodies to HIV, without a positive culture for the virus, or possessing normal
numbers of T-helper lymphocytes are excluded as AIDS cases.

REVISION OF THE CASE DEFINITION

(1) That the case definition of AIDS used for national reporting continue to include only the more severe manifestations of HIV infection

(2) That CDC develop more inclusive definitions and classifications of HIV infection for diagnosis, treatment and prevention, as well as for epidemiologic studies and special surveys

(3) That the following refinements be adopted in the case definition of AIDS used for national reporting.

    (a) In the absence of the opportunistic diseases required by the current case definition, any of the following diseases will be considered indicative of AIDS if the patient has a positive serologic or virologic test for HIV

        (i) Disseminated histoplasmosis (not confined to lungs or lymph nodes), diagnosed by culture, histology, or antigen detection.

        (ii) Isosporiasis, causing chronic diarrhoea (over 1 month), diagnosed by histology or stool microscopy.

        (iii) Bronchial or pulmonary candidiasis, diagnosed by microscopy or by presence of characteristic white plaques grossly on the bronchial mucosa (not by culture alone).

        (iv) Non-Hodgkin's lymphoma of high-grade pathologic type (diffuse, undifferentiated) and of B-cell or unknown immunologic phenotype, diagnosed by biopsy.

        (v) Histologically confirmed Kaposi's sarcoma in patients who are 60 years old or younger when diagnosed.

    (b) In the absence of the opportunistic diseases required by the current case definition, a histologically confirmed diagnosis of chronic lymphoid interstitial pneumonitis in a child (under 13 years of age) will be considered indicative of AIDS unless test(s) for HIV are negative.

    (c) Patients who have a lymphoreticular malignancy diagnosed more than 3 months after the diagnosis of an opportunistic disease used as a marker for AIDS will no longer be excluded as AIDS cases.

(d) To increase the specificity of the case definition, patients will be excluded as AIDS cases if they have a negative result on testing for serum antibody to HIV, have no other type of HIV test with a positive result, and do not have a low number of T-helper lymphocytes or a low ratio of T-helper to T-suppressor lymphocytes. In the absence of test results, patients satisfying all other criteria in the definition will continue to be included.

CASE DEFINITION OF AIDS IN CHILDREN

For the limited purposes of epidemiological surveillance, the CDC define a case of paediatric acquired immune deficiency syndrome (AIDS) as a child who has had:

(1) A reliably diagnosed disease at least moderately indicative of underlying cellular immunodeficiency and

(2) No known cause of underlying cellular immunodeficiency or any other reduced resistance reported to be associated with that disease.

The diseases accepted as sufficiently indicative of underlying cellular immunodeficiency are the same as those used in defining AIDS in adults after the exclusion of congenital infections, e.g. toxoplasmosis or herpes simplex virus infection in the 1st month after birth or cytomegalovirus infection in the first 6 months after birth. A histologically confirmed diagnosis of chronic lymphoid interstitial pneumonitis in a child (under 13 years of age) will be considered indicative of AIDS unless tests for HIV are negative.

Specific conditions that must be excluded in a child are:

(1) Primary immunodeficiency diseases: severe combined immunodeficiency, Di–George syndrome, Wiskott–Aldrich syndrome, ataxia-telangiectasia, graft versus host disease, neutropenia, neutrophil function abnormality, agammaglobulinaemia or hypogammaglobulinaemia with raised IgM.

(2) Secondary immunodeficiency associated with immunosuppressive therapy, lymphoreticular malignancy, or starvation.

General background on viruses

Viruses are the smallest infectious particles known and are a major challenge to medical researchers and clinicians. Some viral infections are mild, self-limiting or asymptomatic. Others, such as rabies and encephalitis, are associated with a high mortality rate. Still others, including the common cold, genital herpes, and influenza have low mortality but high morbidity.

Iwanoski is the 'father' of the science of virology since, in 1892, he recorded the transmission of an infection (tobacco mosaic disease) by an agent which passed freely through a bacteriological filter. Another important milestone for this new discipline was the development of the electron microscope around 1940, which allowed viruses to be seen for the first time. However it was not until 1953 that the Salk inactivated poliovirus vaccine was developed, marking the first major clinical application of modern virology – prophylaxis against a major viral disease.

CHARACTERISTICS OF VIRUSES

Viruses are classified according to their biophysical characteristics:

(1) Presence of nucleic acid – either RNA or DNA
(2) Size
(3) Presence of an envelope
(4) Symmetry – cubic or helical
    Some viruses are naked (e.g. poliovirus) and contain only nucleic

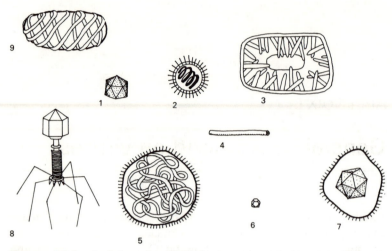

Figure A6.1 1: Adenovirus 2: Influenza virus; 3: Vaccinia virus; 4: Tobacco mosaic virus; 5: Mumps virus; 6: Poliomyelitis virus; 7: Herpes virus; 8: Bacteriophage T_2; 9: Orf virus

acid – either RNA or DNA – and a protein shell, a capsid. Other viruses, such as herpes and influenza, have, in addition, a lipid envelope, acquired during maturation. Since viruses range in size from 17 nm for picornavirus to 300 nm for the poxvirus, they are visible only under electron microscopy.

Morphologically there are three basic forms of viral structure:

(1) Helical viruses, e.g. influenza and mumps
(2) Isometric or icosahedral viruses where the capsid is in the shape of an icosahedron (20 triangular faces and 12 apexes), e.g. herpes and adenovirus
(3) Complex viruses which do not resemble helical or icosahedral, e.g. orf virus

A range of virus structures is shown in Figure A6.1

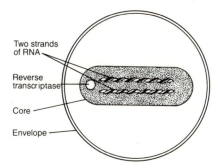

Two strands of RNA

Reverse transcriptase

Core

Envelope

Figure A6.2   Schematic diagram of HIV

STRUCTURE OF THE AIDS VIRUS

The features to note are:

• Envelope or protective coat that shields the core of the virus from the environment
• The presence of the enzyme reverse transcriptase that converts RNA into DNA
• Two strands of RNA

Viruses lack independent metabolism – they reproduce or cause infection only when they are within a host cell. The viral nucleic acid contains all the genetic material necessary for programming the infected host cell to synthesize a number of virus-specific macro-molecules required for viral reproduction. Numerous copies of viral nucleic acid and coat proteins are produced. The capsid encases and stabilizes the viral nucleic acid against its extracellular environment. Upon contact with the new susceptible host cells, the capsid also facilitates the attachment and penetration of the virus. In the target organ, virus multiplication must reach a critical level before cell death occurs and disease becomes obvious.

The multiplication and life cycle of viruses can be described using the example of the reproduction of the bacterial virus T_2 (see Figure A6.3 for details of the events).

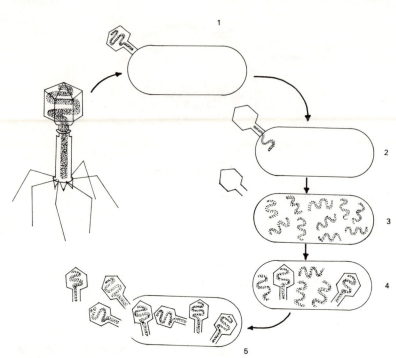

Figure A6.3 Life cycle of a virus (see text)

(1) The virion adsorbs by the tail to a susceptible cell.
(2) The nucleic acid core (DNA) is injected into the bacterial cell.
(3) The viral nucleic acid (DNA) commandeers the bacterial cell to produce viral nucleic acids. This is known as the eclipse phase.
(4) New viral particles are assembled within the bacterial cell. This is known as the rise period.
(5) Swarms of some 200 fully grown viruses escape from the cell. The bacterial cell lyses and dies. This is known as the burst period.

The whole process from start to finish takes only about thirty minutes. In the case of the polio virus in only a few hours a single parasitized cell has produced about 100 000 polio viruses.

The modes of transmission of some human viruses are shown in Table A6.1. With respiratory transmission, infectious viruses implant directly on nasal surfaces from contaminated hands or via droplets

Table A6.1   Modes of transmission of human viruses

Mode of transmission	Symptoms	Viruses
Respiratory (droplets in air, bites, salivary transfer, mouth to hand or object)	Localized	Adenoviruses Rhinoviruses Influenza viruses A, B, C Parainfluenza viruses Coronaviruses
	Generalized	Varicella-zoster; Epstein–Barr (EB) virus Variola (smallpox) Rubella Mumps, measles
Alimentary	Localized	Adenoviruses Enteroviruses Parvoviruses Reoviruses, rotaviruses
	Generalized	Enteroviruses including polioviruses Hepatitis A virus
Contact (skin, mucous membranes)		Wart virus Herpes viruses (herpes simplex virus, type 1 and 2); EB virus Hepatitis B Cytomegalovirus (CMV) Molluscum contagiosum; cowpox
Arthropod bite	Generalized	California encephalitis virus Western equine encephalitis virus Venezuelan equine encephalitis virus
Animal bite	Generalized	Rabies virus
Infection by transfusion	Generalized	HIV Hepatitis B, hepatitis non-A, non-B, EB virus CMV
Transplacental	Generalized	HIV CMV Rubella

from coughs or sneezes. Airborne viruses may enter the lower respiratory passages as well. To reach susceptible cells, virus particles must pass through the mucous film of the nasal epithelium and make physical contact with the cell receptors. The mucus of previously exposed individuals may contain viral inhibitors, such as specific immunoglobulin A (IgA) antibody. However, to induce infection, only a small number of infectious particles need to be implanted in appropriate areas.

Most respiratory viruses cause illness through the direct consequence of local viral multiplication. Subsequent desquamation of the respiratory epithelium is accompanied by necrosis and lysis. Constitutional symptoms may then result from breakdown products of dying cells that are absorbed into the blood stream.

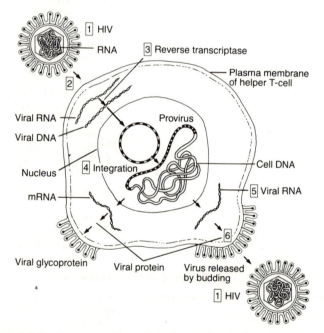

Figure A6.4   Representation of the life cycle of HIV

LIFE CYCLE OF THE AIDS VIRUS

Figure A6.4 shows the life cycle of the AIDS virus – human immunodeficiency virus (HIV). Note the following points:

(1) HIV consists of RNA surrounded by a core of protein which in turn is enclosed in an outer envelope. The envelope is composed of proteins embedded in a lipid bilayer.

(2) Entry of HIV into the helper T-cell is dependent on the interaction of the viral envelope with specific receptors (called T4 receptors) on the T-cell surface.

(3) Once inside the helper T-cell replication of HIV occurs involving the formation of a DNA copy of viral RNA through an enzyme called reverse transcriptase.

(4) The viral DNA then becomes integrated in the host cell DNA.

(5) The DNA then makes viral RNA and messenger RNA. Viral RNA makes up the genetic framework of the newly formed HIV's and messenger RNA makes viral protein – the core and coat of new HIV's.

(6) The immature HIV particles assemble beneath the cell membrane and are released into the bloodstream by a process known as budding.

RESPONSE OF THE HOST

A variety of host responses are activated either in response to natural viral infections or during immunization with live or killed virus. These responses include cellular infiltration, production of humoral and secretory antibodies and activation of cell-mediated immunity. In general, macrophages and a few neutrophils migrate to the inflammatory area. Interferons are produced locally, and B- and T-lymphocytes migrate to infection sites, to the liver, spleen and other organs of the phagocytic system.

Antibodies (Humoral immunity)

Proteins of the virus capsid stimulate B-lymphocytes to synthesize immunoglobulins or humoral antibodies (IgM, IgG, IgD) and a local secretory antibody (IgA), IgE, a mediator of atopic allergies, is also produced.

Antibodies are synthesized throughout the body, in lymph nodes and in inflammatory exudates within the kidney, brain and cervix. The presence of virus-specific IgM indicates a recent infection, as does a fourfold or greater rise in IgG level.

Secretory IgA antibody is manufactured primarily near body surfaces and is found in saliva, colostrum and respiratory secretions. Secretory IgA antibodies in respiratory secretions are vital to the body's defences against respiratory viruses.

Cell-mediated immunity

Cell-mediated immunity is an important defence mechanism against malignant cells and infection from viruses, fungi and some bacteria. It is the most important means of defence against enveloped viruses such as herpes and influenza viruses.

Thymic-derived T-lymphocytes are responsible for cellular immune functions. On initial contact with antigen, the T-cell undergoes clonal proliferation and differentiates into sensitized lymphocytes or 'committed' T-cells with various functions. Some T-lymphocytes become 'activated' and are responsible for mediating cellular immunity. Others become T-memory cells, thereby increasing the number of cells with the ability to react to specific antigen. Still others become helper or suppressor cells and regulate the B-cells' production of antibody.

The 'activated' T-lymphocyte mediates cellular immunity by direct toxic effect, reacting directly with antigens or by releasing chemical mediators called lymphokines. One of these mediators is responsible for markedly augmenting the efficacy of macrophages in inactivating virus.

Endogenous interferons

Within several hours of onset of viral infection and days before humoral antibodies can be measured by ordinary means, antiviral proteins, called interferons, are found in the blood and in tissues in which the virus proliferates. All nucleated cells are capable of producing interferons. Leukocytes produce mostly alfa-interferon; fibroblasts mostly beta-interferon and sensitized T cells, gamma-interferon. In addition to their antiviral activity, interferons are immunoregulatory substances, either stimulator or depressor, depending upon the stage of infection.

Following entry of viral nucleic acid into a susceptible host cell, the cell nucleus is stimulated to produce interferon. Interferon is released through the cytoplasm of the infected cell into the extracellular fluid. It then binds to uninfected cells, activating potent antiviral substances which prevent virus translation and transcription. Interferon has no effect upon extracellular virus, however, which then enters other susceptible cells where the process may be repeated.

DIAGNOSIS OF VIRUS INFECTION

Laboratory procedures used to diagnose viral disease in humans include:

(1) Isolation and identification of virus using cell culture and other techniques.
(2) Measurement of antibodies developing during the course of infection.
(3) Histological examination of infected tissues.
(4) Detection of viral antigens in infected tissue by special techniques involving fluorescein-labelled or peroxidase-labelled antibody.
(5) Electron microscopic examination of vesicular fluids or tissue extracts to identify and count DNA or RNA virus particles.

The method of choice usually depends upon the illness and the availability of specific equipment.

Antibody testing is more readily performed than virus isolation and requires adequately spaced serum samples (usually two to three weeks apart). The diagnosis therefore often is not ellucidated until the patient has either recovered or died. Virus isolation must be attempted when new epidemics occur, or when a specific clinical illness may be caused by many different microorganisms.

Isolation of a virus is not necessarily diagnostic since clinical and epidemiological features consistent with the disease should also be present. Some viruses (e.g. Epstein–Barr or herpes and HIV) may persist for years in the host without causing symptoms. Their presence may be indicative of previous exposure only.

PREVENTION AND TREATMENT OF VIRAL DISEASES

Effective vaccines have been developed for many serious viral diseases, such as hepatitis, influenza, rabies, poliomyelitis, yellow fever, rubella, mumps and measles. The smallpox vaccine has proved so successful that this disease was officially declared eradicated worldwide in 1980.

Immunoglobulins and hyperimmune globulin for certain viral diseases are also available. For example hepatitis B-immune globulin may prevent disease if administered within seven days of exposure. Gamma-globulin is appropriate for use in the prevention of poliomyelitis, measles and hepatitis A in non-immune persons who have been exposed to these diseases.

Since viruses grow only within living cells, researchers face the challenge of discovering antiviral agents which prevent viral replication without interfering with normal cell function. Some antiviral agents are now in widespread use for example acyclovir for herpes and ribavirin for lassa fever.

UK Haemophilia reference centres

Haemophilia Centre,
Coagulation Laboratory
Department of Haematology
St Thomas' Hospital
London SE1 7EH   Tel: 01-928 9292 Ext. 2268

The Katherine Dormandy Haemophilia Centre and Haemostasis Unit
Royal Free Hospital
Pond Street
London NW3 2QG   Tel: 01-794 0500 Ext. 3807

Oxford Haemophilia Centre
Churchill Hospital
Headington
Oxford OX3 7LJ   Tel: 0865 64841 Ext. 532

Department of Clinical Haematology
The Royal Infirmary
Manchester M13 9WL   Tel: 061 273 3300 Ext. 237

Ward P2
Royal Hallamshire Hospital
Glossop Road
Sheffield S10 2JF   Tel: 0742 26484 Ext. 2377

Cardiff Haemophilia Centre
University Hospital of Wales
Heath Park
Cardiff CF4 4XN   Tel: 0222 755944 Ext. 2155

Department of Haematology
Royal Victoria Hospital
Grosvenor Road
Belfast BT12 6BA   Tel: 0232 40503

Department of Haematology
Royal Infirmary
Lauriston Place
Edinburgh   Tel: 031 229 2477 Ext. 2099

Regional Haemophilia Centre
Department of Medicine
Royal Infirmary
Glasgow G4 0SF   Tel: 041 552 3535 Ext. 5127

Haemophilia Centre
The Royal Victoria Infirmary
Queen Victoria Road
Newcastle upon Tyne NE1 4LP   Tel: 0632 325131 Ext. 773

Regional Centres of the National Blood Transfusion Service in the UK

ENGLAND
NORTHERN REGION   Regional Transfusion Centre
                               Westgate Road
                               Newcastle upon Tyne NE4
                                   6QB
                               Tel: 0632 737804/8

YORKSHIRE REGION   Regional Transfusion Centre
                               Bridle Path
                               Leeds LS15 7TW
                               Tel: 0532 645091/3

TRENT REGION   Regional Transfusion Centre
                               Longley Lane
                               Sheffield S5 7JN
                               Tel: 0742 387201

EAST ANGLIAN REGION   Regional Transfusion and
                                   Immuno-haematology
                                   Centre
                               Long Road
                               Cambridge CB2 2PT
                               Tel: 0223 245921

NORTH WEST THAMES
REGION

North London Blood
 Transfusion Centre
Deansbrook Road
Edgware
Middlesex HA8 9BD
Tel: 01-952 5511

NORTH EAST THAMES
REGION

North East Thames Regional
 Transfusion Centre
Crescent Drive
Brentwood
Essex CM15 8DP
Tel: 0277 223545

SOUTH EAST AND
SOUTH WEST THAMES
REGIONS

South London Transfusion
 Centre
75 Cranmer Terrace
London SW17 0RB
Tel: 01-672 8501/7

South London Transfusion
 Sub-Centre
David Salomon's House
Southborough
Nr. Tonbridge
Kent
Tel: 0892 28172

WESSEX REGION

Wessex Regional Transfusion
 Centre
Coxford Road
Southampton SO9 5UP
Tel: 0703 776441

OXFORD REGION

Regional Transfusion Centre
John Radcliffe Hospital
Headington
Oxford OX3 7LJ
Tel: 0865 65711

SOUTH WESTERN
REGION

South West Regional
 Transfusion Centre
Southmead Road
Bristol BS10 5ND
Tel: 0272 507777

WEST MIDLANDS
REGION

Regional Transfusion Centre
Vincent Drive
Edgbaston
Birmingham B15 2SG
Tel: 021 472 3111

MERSEY REGION

Regional Blood Transfusion
    Centre
West Derby Street
Mount Vernon
Liverpool L7 8TW
Tel: 051 709 7272

NORTH WESTERN
REGION

Regional Transfusion Centre
Plymouth Grove
Manchester M13 9LL
Tel: 061 273 7181

Transfusion Centre
Quernmore Road
Lancaster LA1 3JP
Tel: 0524 63456

WALES

Regional Transfusion Centre
Rhyd-Lafar
St Fagans
Cardiff CF5 6XF
Tel: 0222 890302

SCOTLAND

North of Scotland Blood
    Transfusion Service
Raigmore Hospital
Inverness IV2 3UJ
Tel: 0463 34151

Aberdeen and North-East
    Scotland Blood Transfusion
    Service
Royal Infirmary
Foresterhill
Aberdeen AB9 2ZW
Tel: 0224 681818 Ext. 2086

East of Scotland Blood
    Transfusion Service
Ninewells Hospital
Dundee DD1 9SY
Tel: 0382 645166

Edinburgh and South-East
    Scotland Blood Transfusion
    Service
Royal Infirmary
Edinburgh EH3 9HB
Tel: 031 229 2585

Glasgow and West of
   Scotland Blood Transfusion
   Service
Law Hospital
Carluke
Lanarkshire ML8 5ES
Tel: 0698 373315

Scottish National Blood
   Transfusion Service
Headquarters Office
Ellen's Glen Road
Edinburgh EH17 7QT
Tel: 031 664 2317

NORTHERN IRELAND

Blood Transfusion Service
89 Durham Street
Belfast BT12 4GE
Tel: 0232 46464

APPENDIX 8

Selected Bibliography and Useful Addresses

(1) The following are recommended for general background reading – the publications are free unless otherwise stated

  (i) AIDS and Employment
    The Mailing House
    Leeland Road
    London
    W13 9HL

      ● *AIDS and Employment*

  (ii) AVERT
    (AIDS Virus Education and Research Trust)
    PO Box 91
    Horsham
    West Sussex
    RH13 7YR

      ● *AIDS is everyone's problem*

  (iii) COHSE
    (Confederation of Health Service Employees)
    Glen House
    High Street
    Banstead
    Surrey
    Tel: Burgh Heath (07373) 53322

      ● *AIDS – guidelines for health staffs dealing with patients suffering from Acquired Immune Deficiency Syndrome or with AIDS virus* (Price £2)

  (iv) The Department of Health and Social Security AIDS unit
    Alexander Fleming House
    Elephant and Castle
    London
    SE1 6BY
    Tel: 01–403 1893

    Documents from:
    DHSS Store
    Health Publications Unit
    No. 2 Site
    Manchester Road
    Heywood
    Lancs. OL10 2PZ

      ● *AIDS – General Information for Doctors –* 15 pages, May 1985.
      ● *AIDS – Booklet 2: Information for Doctors Concerning the Introduction of the HTLV III Antibody –* 12 pages, October 1985.

- *AIDS Booklet 3: Guidance for Surgeons, Anaesthetists, Dentists and their teams in dealing with patients infected with HTLV III –* April 1986.
- *Children at school and problems related to AIDS –* DES Administrative Memorandum 2/86. CMO (86) 10: June 1986.
- *DHSS – Information and guidance on AIDS for local authority staff –* (LASSL 86/8), 8 pages, July 23, 1986.
- *Acquired Immune Deficiency Syndrome (AIDS) and Artificial Insemination – Guidance for Doctors and AI Clinics –* CMO (86) 12: July 1986.
- *Advisory Committee on Dangerous Pathogens – LAV/HTLV III – the causative agent of AIDS and related conditions.* Revised guidelines, 30 pages, June 1986.

(v) The Gay Medical Association
BM/GMA
London
WC1N 3XX

(vi) The Haemophilia Society
123 Westminster Bridge Road
London
SE1 7HR
Tel: 01–928 2020

- *Haemofact*
- *AIDS and the blood* (booklet – price £2)

(vii) The Health Education Council
78 New Oxford Street
London
WC1A 1AH
Tel: 01–631 0930

- *Guide to a healthy sex life*
- *Some Facts About AIDS*
- *AIDS: What everybody needs to know*

(viii) The Health and Safety Executive
Library and Information Service
Baynards House
1 Chepstow Place
Westbourne Grove
London
W2 4TF
Tel: 01–221 0416

- *Safety in health service laboratories: labelling, transport and reception of specimens*

(ix) National Association of Citizens Advice Bureaux
115–123 Pentonville Road
London
N1 9LZ
Tel: 01–833 2181

- *Briefing to help bureau staff who get involved in counselling people with AIDS*

(x) The National Blood Transfusion Service
North London Blood Transfusion Centre
Deansbrook Road
Edgware
Middlesex
HA8 9BD
Tel: 01–952 5511

- *AIDS – What you must know before you give blood*

(xi) The National Union of
Students
461 Holloway Road
London N7 6LJ
Tel: 01–272 8900

● *AIDS – the facts*

(xii) The Public Relations
Department
NW Thames Regional
Health Authority
40 Eastbourne Terrace
London
W2 3QR
Tel: 01–262 8011 Ext. 324

● *AIDS – the St Mary's
Control of Infection Pack*
(Price £6)

(xiii) Royal College of Nursing
RCN Publications
Department
20 Cavendish Square
London
W1M 0AB
Tel: 01–409 3333

● *Guidelines for the
management of AIDS
patients both in hospital and
the community* (price £1.80)

(xiv) SCODA
(Standing Conference On
Drug Abuse)
1–4 Hatton Place
Hatton Garden
London
EC1N 8ND
Tel: 01–430 2341/2

● *AIDS – How Drug Users
Can Avoid It*

(xv) The Terrence Higgins Trust
BM AIDS
London
WC1N 3XX
Tel: 01–833 2971

● *AIDS – a medical briefing*
● *AIDS – the facts*
● *AIDS – more facts for gay
men*
● *AIDS HTLV III Antibody;
To test or not to test?*
● *Facts about AIDS for Drug
Users*
● *SEX*
● *Women and AIDS*
● *Is it safe – the chalice and
AIDS*

(xvi) Thames Television
'Help Programme'
149 Tottenham Court Road
London
W1 9LL
Tel: 01–387 9494

● *The facts about AIDS*

(xvii) Women's Reproductive
Rights Information Centre
52–54 Featherstone Street
London
EC1Y 8RT
Tel: 01–251 6332

● *Women and AIDS*

(2) Books/Publications

Altman, D. (1986) *AIDS and the New Puritanism*. Pluto Press, £4.95

Cahill, K. M. (1984) *The AIDS Epidemic*. Hutchinson, £3.95

Daniels, V. G. (1986) *AIDS – Questions and Answers*. Cambridge Medical Books, £3.75

Devita, V. T. *et al.* (Eds) (1985) *AIDS, Aetiology, Diagnosis, Treatment and Prevention*. J. B. Lippincott Co., £49.50

Farthing, C. *et al.* (1986) *A Colour Atlas of AIDS*. Wolfe Medical Publications, £12.00

Gong, V. (Ed.) (1985) *Understanding AIDS: A Comprehensive Guide*. Cambridge University Press, £19.50

Green, J. and Miller, D. (1986) *AIDS: The Story of a Disease*. Grafton Books, £5.95

Greenspan, D. *et al.* (1986) *AIDS and the Dental Team*. Munksgaard, £10.00

Hancock, G. (1986) *AIDS the Deadly Epidemic*. Gollancz, £3.95

Jones, P. (1985) *AIDS and the Blood: A Practical Guide*. Haemophilia Society, £2.00

Jones, P. (Ed.) (1986) *Proceedings of the AIDS Conference*. Intercept, £12.50

Mayer, K. & Pizer, H. (1983) *The AIDS Fact Book*. Bantam Books, £2.75

Miller, D. *et al.* (Eds) (1986) *The Management of AIDS Patients*. Macmillan, £9.95

Pratt, R. J. (1986) *AIDS: A Strategy for Nursing Care*. Edward Arnold, £6.75

Royal College of Nursing (1986) *AIDS Nursing Guidelines*. RCN, £3.75

Tatchell, P. (1986) *Surviving the AIDS Crisis*. Gay Men's Press, £2.95

Vass, A. A. (1986) *AIDS: A Plague On Us – A Social Perspective*. Venus Academica, £7.95

Weber, J. and Ferriman, F. A. (1986) *AIDS Concerns You*. Pagoda Books, £2.95

The Bureau of Hygiene and Tropical Diseases, Keppel Street, London WC1E 7HT 01–636–8636, produce several excellent publications on AIDS (prices on application)

  (i) *AIDS Newsletter* (produced 20 times a year)
  (ii) *AIDS and retroviruses update* (abstracting service)
  (iii) *Abstracts on Hygiene and Communicable Diseases*
  (iv) An AIDS Database on DataStar, BRS Information Technologies and CAB International.

AIDS videos

(a) *AIDS: The Reality and the Myth.* Master Class Video. Running time
    42 mins., £19.95, available from Cambridge Medical Books, Tracey
    Hall, Cockburn Street, Cambridge CB1 3NB. Tel: 0223 212423

(b) *'You Can't Catch AIDS by ...'* £23, available from Film and
    Television Unit, Royal Society of Medicine, 1 Wimpole Street,
    London W1M 8AE

(3) Useful addresses and telephone numbers – UK

(a) Terrence Higgins Trust
    BM AIDS,
    LONDON
    WC1N 3XX
    Telephone: 01–833 2971
    Monday to Friday 7 pm–
    10 pm
    Saturday and Sunday
    3 pm–10 pm

(b) Haemophilia Society
    123 Westminster Bridge
    Road
    LONDON
    SE1 7HR
    Telephone: 01–428 2020

(c) Health Education Council
    78 New Oxford Street,
    LONDON
    WC1
    Telephone: 01–637 1881

(d) SCODA (Standing
    Conference on Drug
    Abuse)
    1–4 Hatton Place
    LONDON
    EC1N 8ND
    Telephone: 01–430 2341

(e) Healthline Telephone
    Service
    01–981 2717
    01–980 7222
    From outside London 0345
    581151

(f) Gay Switchboard
    BM Switchboard,
    LONDON
    WC1N 3XX
    Telephone: 01–837 7324

(g) London Friend
    274 Upper Street,
    LONDON
    N1
    Telephone: 01–359 7371

(h) Publications which carry
    regular articles about
    AIDS. Contact the
    publishers directly.
    Capital Gay   01–273 3766
    Gay News   01–995 3335
    Gay Times   01–267 2164
    Out   01–740 9200

(i) Gay Bereavement Project
    46 Wentworth Road
    LONDON
    NW11 0RL

(j) Christian Action on AIDS
    47 Venns Lane
    HEREFORD
    Telephone: 0432 268167

(4) AIDS/HIV support groups

The list is by no means exhaustive, and if a group is not listed for your area or region, check with your local genito-urinary medicine clinic (STD) which may have knowledge of local groups.

East Anglia Region
Cambridge AIDS Help Group,
P.O. Box 257,
Cambridge CB2 1XQ.
Telephone: 0223 69765.

Mersey Region
Merseyside AIDS Support Group,
63 Shamrock Road, Birkenhead,
Merseyside L41 0EG.
Telephone line: 051 7080234. Wed 7-10 pm.

Northern Region
AIDS North,
P O Box 1BD,
Newcastle Upon Tyne NE99 1BB.

Northern Ireland
Cara-friend,
P O Box 44,
Belfast BT1 1SH.
Telephone lines: Belfast 222023. Mon-Thurs 7.30 pm-10.00 pm.
Londonderry   263120.   Thurs 7.30 pm-10.00 pm.

North Western Region
Manchester AIDS Line,
P O Box 201,
Manchester M60 1PU.
Telephone line: 061 2281617. Mon, Wed, Fri 7-10 pm.

Oxford Region
OXAIDS, c/o Harrison Department,
Radcliffe Infirmary,
Oxford.
Telephone line: 0865 246036. Wed 6-8 pm.

Oxford Body Positive,
Freepost, Nether Westcote,
Oxford OX7 6BR.
Telephone line: 0865 246036.

Reading Area AIDS Support Group,
P O Box 75, Reading,
Berkshire.
Telephone line: 0734 503377. Thurs 8-10 pm.

Milton Keynes AIDS Support Group,
P O Box 153, Wolverton,
Milton Keynes.
Telephone line: 0908 312196. Mon 7-9 pm.

Scotland
Scottish AIDS Monitor,
P O Box 169,
Edinburgh, Scotland.
Telephone line: 031 5581167. Tues 7-10 pm (ansaphone at other times).

AIDS Information and Counselling Service,
129 Kilmarnock Road,
Shawlands, Glasgow G41 3YT.

South Western Region
Aled Richards Trust,
2 Cliftonwood Crescent,
Cliftonwood, Bristol BS8 4TU.
Telephone line: 0272 276436. Thurs 7-10 pm.

Thames Regions
North East Thames
Camden AIDS,
Area Three Social Services,
West End Lane, London NW6.

PASAC, P O Box 130,
Colchester, Essex.
Telephone line: 0206 560225. Mon,
Wed 7-9 pm.

North West Thames
Bedford Gay Helpline,
58 Cherry Walk, Kempston,
Bedford.

South East Thames
Medway and Maidstone Gay
  Switchboard,
P O Box 10C,
Chatham, Kent ME4 6TX.
Telephone line: 0634 826925.
Thurs/Fri 7.30-9 pm.

Sussex AIDS Helpline,
P O Box 17, Brighton BN2 5NQ.
Telephone line: 0273 734316. Mon-
Fri 8-10 pm.

South West Thames
CALM, P O Box 11,
Bognor Regis, West Sussex PO21
  1AH.
Telephone line: 0243 776998. Mon,
Wed, Fri 7-9.30 pm.

Trent Region
Nottingham AIDS Info Group,
Sharespace, 49 Stoney Street,
Nottingham.
Telephone line: 0602 585526. Mon,
Tues 7-10 pm.

Wessex Region
Bournemouth AIDS Support
  Group,
P O Box 263,
Bournemouth BH8 8DY.
Telephone line: 0202 38850. Mon,
Tues 8-10 pm.

Solent AIDS Line,
P O Box 139,
Southampton, Hants.
Telephone line: 0703 37363. Tues,
Thurs, Sat 7.30-10 pm.

West Midlands
AIDS Concern Midlands,
79 Stanmore Road,
Edgbaston, Birmingham B16 9SU.
Telephone line: 021 6221511. Tues
7.30-9.30 pm.

Yorkshire Region
Bradford Gay Switchboard Col-
  lective,
643 Littlehalton Lane,
Bradford BD5 8BY.
Telephone line: 0274 42895. Sun,
Tues, Thurs 7-9 pm.

Leeds AIDS Information and Counselling Service,
11 Plaintree View,
Shadwell, Leeds 17.

Leeds AIDS Line,
64-68 Call Lane,
Leeds LS2.
Telephone line: 0532 441661. Tues
7-9 pm.

West Yorkshire AIDS Support
  Group,
1 Cambridge Street,
Hebdon Bridge, West Yorkshire
HX7 6LN.

Irish Republic
Gay Health Action,
10 Fownes Street,
Dublin 2, Eire.
Telephone line: Dublin 710939.
Mon-Fri 11 am-4 pm.

(5) AIDS organizations – USA

Gay Rights National Lobby
Box 1892
Washington, DC 20013
(202) 546-1801

KS Research and Education Foundation
54 Tenth Street
San Francisco, CA 94103
(415) 864-4376

National Coalition of Gay STD Services
P O Box 239
Milwaukee, WI 53201
(414) 277-7671

National Gay Task Force
80 Fifth Avenue – Suite 1601
New York, NY 10011
(212) 741-5800
Crisisline: 1-800-221-7044
(212) 807-6016 (New York, Alaska, Hawaii)

Public Health Service
Department of Health and Human Services
Washington, DC 20201
(202) 245-6867

California

Los Angeles
KS Foundation/Los Angeles
Gay/Lesbian Community Center
1213 North Highland Avenue
Los Angeles, CA 90038
(213) 461-1333

L.A. AIDS Project
937 W. Cole Street – Suite 3
Los Angeles, CA 90038
(213) 871-2437 (Hotline)
(213) 871-1284 (Office)

L.A. Sex Information Hotline
8405 Beverly Boulevard
Los Angeles, CA 90048
(213) 653-2118

Southern California Physicians for Human Rights
7985 Santa Monica Boulevard – Suite 109
165
Los Angeles, CA
(213) 658-6261 (Business)
(213) 860-6611

Sacramento
AIDS & KS Foundation/Sacramento
2115 J Street – Suite # 3
Sacramento, CA 95816
(916) 448-AIDS

Beach Area Community Clinic
3705 Mission Blvd.
San Diego, CA 92109
(619) 488-0644

Owen Clinic
University of California
San Diego Medical Center
225 Dickinson Street
San Diego, CA 92103
(619) 294-3995

San Francisco
American Association of Physicians for Human Rights
P.O. Box 14366
San Francisco, CA 94114
(415) 673-3189

Bay Area Physicians for Human Rights
P.O. Box 14546
San Francisco, CA 94114
(415) 558-9353 (Administration)
(415) 372-7321 (Medical inquiries)

Kaposi's Sarcoma Clinic
University of California, San Francisco
Medical Center, A-312
San Francisco, CA 94143
(415) 666-1407

KS Research and Education Foundation
54 Tenth Street
San Francisco, CA 94103
(415) 864-4376

Shanti Project
890 Hayes Street
San Francisco, CA 94117
(415) 558-9644

Colorado

Colorado AIDS Project
Gay and Lesbian Community Center
1436 Lafayette Street
Denver, CO 80218
(303) 831-6268

Gay and Lesbian Health Alliance
P.O. Box 6101
Denver, CO 80206
(303) 777-9530

Connecticut

AIDS Project/New Haven
Box 7
North Haven, CT 06473
(203) 239-7881

Hartford Gay Health Collective
320 Farmington Avenue
Hartford, CT 06105
(203) 527-9813

Yale Self-Care Network
17 Hillhouse Avenue
New Haven, CT 06520

Delaware

G.L.A.D.
P.O. Box 9218
Wilmington, DE 19809
1-800-342-4012
(302) 764-2208

District of Columbia

Whitman-Walker Clinic
2335 18th Street, NW
Washington, DC 20009
(202) 332-5295

Florida

Miami
AIDS Support Group
c/o MCC Church
23rd St & NE 2nd St
Miami, FL
(305) 573-4156

University of Miami Medical School
AIDS Project
Department of Medicine R-42
Miami, FL
(305) 325-6338

Tampa
University of South Florida
Main Lab, Medical Clinic S.
12901 North 30th Street
Tampa, Fl 33612
(813) 974-4214

Key West
AIDS Action Committee
Florida Keys Memorial Hospital
P.O. Box 4073
Key West, FL 33041

Monroe County Health Dept
Public Service Building
Junior College Road
Key West, FL 33040
(305) 294-1021

Georgia

AID Atlanta
1801 Piedmont Road
Atlanta, GA 30324
(404) 872-0600

Centers for Disease Control
AIDS Activity
Building 3, Room 5B-1
1600 Clifton Road
Atlanta, GA 30333
(404) 329-3472

Illinois

Howard Brown Memorial Clinic
AIDS Action
2676 N. Halstead Street
Chicago, IL 60614
(312) 871-5777 (Office/Medical)
(312) 871-5776 (Hotline)

Louisiana

Crescent City Coalition
c/o St Louis Community Center
1022 Barracks Street
New Orleans, LA 70116
(504) 568-9619

Maryland

AIDS Hotline
101 W. Read Street – Suite 815
Baltimore, MD 21201
(301) 244-8484 (Medical Office)
(301) 947-2437

Gay Community Center Clinic
241 W. Chase Street
Baltimore, MD 21201
(301) 837-2050

Massachusetts

Boston Department of Health
AIDS Hotline
(617) 424-5916

Fenway Community Health Center,
   or AIDS Action Committee
16 Haviland Street
Boston, MA 02215
(617) 267-7573

Mayor's Ad Hoc Committee on
   AIDS
c/o Boston City Hall – Room 608
Boston, MA 02201
(617) 725-4849

Minnesota

AIDS Support Group
c/o 2309 Girard Ave. South
Minneapolis, MN 55405

Minnesota AIDS Project
c/o Lesbian & Gay Community Services
124 W. Lake St – Suite E
Minneapolis, MN 55408

New Hampshire

New Hampshire Feminist Health
   Center
232 Court Street
Portsmouth, NH 03801
(603) 436-6171

New Jersey
New Jersey Lesbian and Gay AIDS
   Awareness
c/o St Michaels Medical Center
268 High Street
Newark, NJ 07102
(201) 596-0767

New York

Gay Men's Health Crisis
P.O. Box 274
132 W. 24th Street
New York, NY 10011
(212) 685-4952
(212) 807-6655

Gay Men's Health Project
74 Grove Street – # 2J
New York, NY 10014
(212) 691-6969

New York City Department of Health
Office of Gay and Lesbian Health Concerns
125 Worth Street – # 806
New York, NY 10013
(212) 566-6110

St Mark's Clinic
88 University Place
New York, NY 10003
(212) 691-8282

Ohio

Cincinnati
Ambrose Clement Health Clinic
STD Clinic
3101 Burnet Avenue
Cincinnati, OH 45229
(513) 352-3143

Cleveland
Cleveland Health Issues
11800 Edgewater Street, # 206
Lakewood, OH 44107
(216) 822-7285 (Daytime)
(216) 266-6507 (After 6 pm)

Free Medical Clinic of Greater Cleveland
12201 Euclid Avenue
Cleveland, OH 44106
(216) 721-4010

Oklahoma

Oklahoma Blood Institute
1001 Lincoln Boulevard
Oklahoma City, OK
(405) 239-2437

Oklahomans for Human Rights
1932 'C' South Cheyenne Street
Tulsa, OK 74119
(918) 583-7323

Oregon

Phoenix Rising/Cascade AIDS Project
408 Southwest 2nd Ave. – Room 403
Portland, OR 97204
(503) 223-8299

Pennsylvania

Philadelphia
AIDS Task Force
c/o Philadelphia City Health Department
P.O. Box 7529
Philadelphia, PA 19101
(215) 574-9666 (Office)
(215) 232-8055 (Hotline)

Philadelphia Community Health Alternatives
P.O. Box 7259
Philadelphia, PA 19109
(215) 624-2879

Pittsburgh
Graduate School of Public Health
University of Pittsburgh Health Center
A-417 Crabtree Hall
Pittsburgh, PA 15261
(412) 624-3928
(412) 624-3331

Texas

Dallas
AIDS Action Project
c/o Oaklawn Counselling Center
Suite 202
3409 Oaklawn Street
Dallas, TX 75219
(214) 528-2181

Houston
KS/AIDS Foundation of Houston
3317 Montrose Boulevard
Houston, TX 77006
(713) 524-2437

The Montrose Clinic
104 Westheimer
Houston, TX 77006
(713) 528-5531
(713) 528-5535

San Antonio
Safeweek/AIDS Committee
1713 West Mulberry
San Antonio, TX 78201
(512) 736-5216

Washington

Gay Men's Health Group
2353 Minor Ave. E.
Seattle, WA 98102
(206) 322-3919

Harbor View Medical Center
STD Clinic
324 9th – ZA-85
Seattle, WA 98104
(206) 223-3000

NW AIDS Foundation
P.O. Box 3449
Seattle, WA 98114
(206) 527-8770
(206) 622-9650

Wisconsin

Madison
Blue Bus Clinic
1552 University Avenue
Madison, WI 53706
(608) 262-7440

Milwaukee
Brady East STD Clinic
1240 East Brady Street
Milwaukee, WI 53202
(414) 272-2144

National Coalition of Gay Sexually
   Transmitted   Disease   Services
   (NCGSTDS)
P.O. Box 239
Milwaukee, WI 53201

Index